THE HEALING MAGIC OF

forest bathing

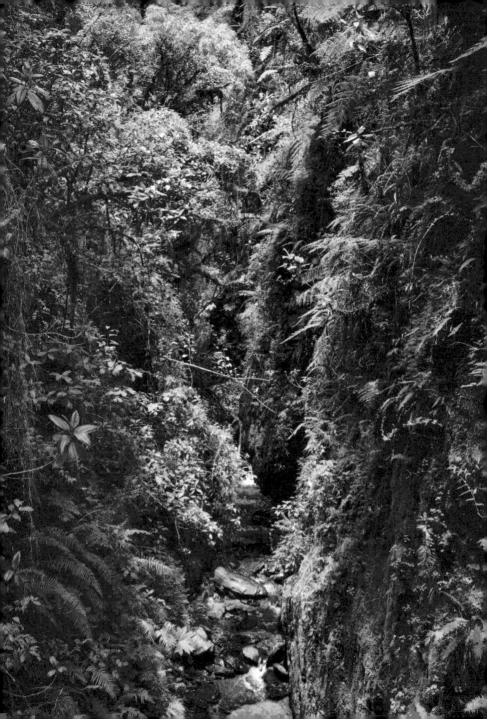

THE HEALING MAGIC OF

forest bathing

Finding Calm, Creativity,
and Connection in the Natural World

JULIA PLEVIN

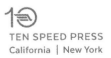

TEN SPEED PRESS
California | New York

Contents

1   INTRODUCTION

5   PART 1
BEGIN THE JOURNEY
TO RECONNECTION

- 6   Live Your Life
- 13   From Haiku to *Shinrin-yoku*
- 18   Welcome to the New Environmental Movement
- 22   Forest Bathing Is a Way of Life

25   PART 2
HEED THE CALL
OF THE FOREST

- 26   Prepare for the Journey
- 33   Get Outside and Find a Place
- 36   Show Up
- 38   Shake Off the Road Dust
- 41   Disconnect to Reconnect
- 43   Practice Presence
- 45   Set an Intention
- 48   Get Lost in Space

51   PART 3
CROSS THE THRESHOLD

- 52   Say a Prayer for the Forest
- 54   Tread Lightly
- 57   Give Offerings
- 59   Ask Permission
- 61   Cultivate Tree Energy
- 63   Connect with a Tree
- 65   Greet the Sun

69   PART 4
MOVE THROUGH
INVITATIONS

- 70   Walk in Silence
- 72   Find Yourself in Fractals
- 75   Come to Your Senses
- 79   Bathe in the Benefits
- 83   Look Up
- 84   Let It Go
- 86   Find Your Rhythm
- 88   Sing with the Land

90 Get Elemental

94 Converse with Trees

97 Sit in a Sacred Spot

100 Eat a Snack

105 Spark Your Creativity

108 Take a Nap

111 Host a Ceremony

115 **PART 5**
FIND YOUR TRUE NATURE

116 Love Yourself

119 Follow Your Heart

123 Notice Signposts and
Guideposts

127 Hear What the Earth
Wants to Tell You

130 Discover Your Own Medicine

135 **PART 6**
RETURN WITH YOUR ELIXIR

136 Thank the Forest

138 Take Time to Reflect

140 Keep the Connection Alive

143 Share Nutrients

145 Designate a Prayer Tree

147 Honor the Old-Growth

151 Heal the Planet

154 **FURTHER READING**

156 **ENDNOTES**

163 **SPECIAL THANKS**

165 **ABOUT THE AUTHOR**

166 **INDEX**

TO ALL THOSE WHO HAVE ENTERED
THE FOREST BEFORE ME AND WITH
ME, AND THOSE WHO WILL COME
AFTER ME. FOR MOTHER EARTH
AND ALL HER INHABITANTS.

Introduction

However this book got to you, the fact that you're reading it now means that you're ready to embark on your own journey of reconnection. There's no more time to waste and no room for excuses. Now is the time to begin. This book is about what forest bathing is, how it came to be, and why we all need it now more than ever. Your journey starts when you step into the forest. You're invited.

"Go out in the woods, go out. If you don't go out in the woods nothing will ever happen and your life will never begin."

—CLARISSA PINKOLA ESTÉS, *Women Who Run with the Wolves*

HOW TO USE THIS BOOK

My intention in writing this book is to open the door to the world of *interbeing*—the essential connectedness of the Universe—and then get out of your way. I'm here to witness your journey and walk alongside you. Your story will be different from my story: we each get to have our own perfectly designed experience. Yours is waiting for you.

As you read, you'll learn about the forest bathing journey. The sections of this book mirror the structure of a forest bath, from preparing for the journey in the beginning to integrating the elixir of the forest behaviors so we can reacquaint with our true selves and, with that, the web that comprises every living thing. Everywhere, forests are vying for our attention. They desire to be seen and noticed and will do everything in their power to get us to slow down and wake up to life. Forests and trees call to all of us; they need our help as much as we need theirs. We can save one another. That longing in your heart to go to the forest is real.

You may start with a trip to a forest, but true forest bathing extends into rituals and practices that you will eventually incorporate into your everyday life. A forest bath is not a "one and done" kind of experience. And there's no right or wrong way to forest bathe; it's a personal experience in which each of us finds what works best.

Begin with the intention of reconnecting to Nature and the realization that you're separated from the source; the life you desire for yourself is on the other side of the separation. In the process, you'll relearn some of the basic tenets of being a human—like how to walk, how to breathe, how to open your heart, and how to be truly present.

No two forest baths are the same. When you go into the forest, you may get the forest bath you need instead of the one you want. Forest bathing involves no specific time requirements. On some days, you may have time to spend a few hours immersed in nature. Other days, you may only have a few sacred moments to connect. You can forest bathe time and again, and each visit will be different. There are infinite activations and ways to connect—you'll discover what works best for you. Trust that the forest is working alongside you to design the perfect experience.

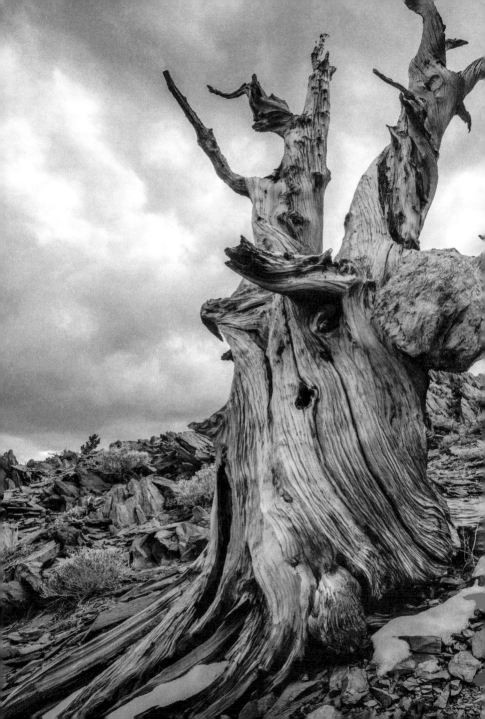

PART 1

BEGIN THE JOURNEY TO RECONNECTION

The most important and fulfilling work we as humans can do on this planet at this time is to reconnect to ourselves, to one another, and to the natural world. All of the best stories of reconnection start in the same place: a state of total despair. The journey begins before you're totally aware of it. The call to return to nature—your true nature—comes from deep inside and often manifests as chaos in life before you really begin to pay attention. If you slow down and take a moment to listen, you might hear the call before it intensifies. This is the way of forest bathing.

live your life

It sounds dramatic, but it's true: forest bathing saved my life Through forest bathing, I've learned to live my own true life instead of the life I thought I was expected to live, based on where I came from, what my parents or peers expected from me, where I went to school and what I studied, or any other way we all end up living someone else's life.

They say that the medicine you have to offer is the medicine that you need. The medicine I need is definitely forest bathing. And I take my medicine every day.

I'm a highly sensitive person and have experienced periods of inexplicable illness, intense anxiety, and debilitating depression. I first found my way to forest bathing while in design school in New York City. I had always been outdoorsy and felt best when hiking, surfing, climbing, or just adventuring in the great wild, but it wasn't until I was living in Brooklyn and going to school in Manhattan that the lack of nature in my life became an all-encompassing itch that I could not scratch. So I chose to focus my entire graduate thesis on psychoterratica—the mental health effects of being disconnected from nature. It started as an academic pursuit, but as I read the research, I began to see myself reflected on those pages.

I've known that I am affected by seasonal affective disorder (SAD) since my time at Dartmouth College. And I am not alone: studies show that the lack of light resulting from winter darkness affects, to some degree, about 20 percent of the US population.[1] But SAD isn't the only way we are affected by nature: the lack of connection to nature is the root cause of much of our mental and emotional distress.

I thought I would feel better once I left the monochrome gray of New York City and moved west to sunny California, but of course my issues came with me across the country. I was trying my hardest to keep up the semblance of having it all together amidst dealing with confusing health issues and bouts of anxiety and depression, a failing relationship, paying off exorbitant student loans, and searching for a job. Finally, I got worn down to the point where I couldn't hold all the pieces of life together. I simply gave up. And in giving up, I gave in. Little did I know that life really begins once we give up trying to control it—at least that's what happened for me.

I'm an avid runner and used to be in such a rush all the time. I had been running through life like a race, as though there was a finish line and I had to get there first. I would actually *run* my errands with shopping bags, because walking took too long. For years, the only time I spent in the forest was while running through on trails.

Then, during one run in Mount Sutro Forest, an urban forest on the western side of San Francisco, a man stopped me.

"Hey! Do you know why there are ribbons around these trees?" he asked.

"No," I said, rushing by. "I just moved back here! It's my first time here in years." I didn't like being stopped. But he kept talking. He told me the trees were being cut down and asked me to look at a website, sutroforest.com, to learn more about what was happening there.

I was in a state of distress throughout the rest of my run. When I looked at the website after returning home, I was aghast. How could a forest in the middle of a city as eco-conscious as San Francisco be in danger of being cut down? Who else even knew about this? I resolved to do everything in my power to protect this special place.

What I didn't realize then was that the Mount Sutro Forest was calling to me. The forest needed help. It took some man literally stopping me in my tracks to get me to slow down, get out of my own head, and notice what was happening around me. I believe he must have been sent from the Universe to give me a message that I was just missing time and time again. If not for him, I'd probably still be running on that treadmill of life.

I had finished my graduate work but was just beginning the real work. I began to understand that connecting to Nature was the cure for all the ways that being disconnected from it makes us sick. It was almost too simple and obvious to be true. I surrendered to the call of the forest. As I began a practice of communing with Nature with the intention to heal and connect on a deeper level, something magical, beyond logic, started to happen. My life began to expand and unfold in ways I had never imagined. The anxiety, stress, and fear that had been keeping me small and sick subsided, and I slowly began to trust in the natural unfolding of my life, the way a fern trusts its own unfurling.

Every time I mentioned forest bathing in conversation, people would get this dreamy look in their eyes. "I want that!" they'd tell me, even if they weren't totally sure what forest bathing was. It was like they desired it on a subconscious level. And now, after facilitating forest baths

"It is easier to live through someone else than to complete yourself. The freedom to lead and plan your own life is frightening if you have never faced it before. It is frightening when a woman finally realizes that there is no answer to the question 'who am I' except the voice inside herself."

—BETTY FRIEDAN, *The Feminine Mystique*

for hundreds of people, I can attest to its importance as a universal practice. No one ever says, "Nature? Nah. Not for me." No matter who we are, what we look like, or where we've been—we all come from nature. Nature is home to each of us, and forest bathing is a walk home.

I created the Forest Bathing Club on meetup.com just to see if anyone would want to join me on excursions into the forest. I started the club because *I* needed it to exist. Within a few months, the group had grown to more than five hundred people, and journalists from far and wide were covering forest baths like it was breaking news! Soon, people who had been doing this type of work for decades started to appear out of the blue sky to show me how to further my own practice. And I started to feel called to certain places and people who were also on this journey of reconnection.

There's no logical explanation for how the club gained so much momentum so fast, but I knew it was beyond me. I realized that I had tapped into something bigger than myself, something better designed than I could design. I was designing alongside the best designer of them all—Mother Earth. I had a sense that I was doing the work I was put on this planet at this time to do, and the forest spirits were propelling the work forward. Whenever I would get anxious or stressed, I would find ways to reconnect with Nature and receive reassurance that as long as I was doing this important work and sharing it with as many people as I could, I would be supported.

Each time I go into the forest, I learn something new and integrate it into my forest bathing practice. I created a process that lets me come to presence, quiet my mind, release my fears, and call in my true desires. With every visit to the forest, I discover things that no one has ever taught me—that I can have a conversation with the trees, sing with the plants, and share messages with the birds. I said to Nature, "Teach me! Teach me!" and she did. I discovered books and blogs on the far-flung corners of the internet, with titillating teachings on the vast subject of connecting to Nature. Nature speaks to us through a knowing in our hearts, and the heart chakra's corresponding color is green. The more time we spend among trees and plants, the stronger we feel the connection between our hearts and the world.

I went into the forest tentatively at first, unsure of how I was supposed to act. Over time, I grew more comfortable there, and now I scream and dance. I sing to the forest, give it offerings, and treasure its ever-changing landscapes. I give high fives to ferns when I'm happy and cry under the willows when I'm sad. I lose myself in the intricacies of the patterns of a fallen leaf and completely surrender to the awe-inspiring beauty of the redwoods. I make bouquets of leaves, twirl sticks, and look for shapes in the clouds. I express and live out my feelings and emotions so that I can be in a fluid exchange of energy with Earth and not get clogged up and confused.

Since that fated run during a tough transition, my entire life has been transformed. The dreams that I had been too afraid to dream for myself began to come true, and as they did, I began to trust that my dreams and visions were leading the way. I have followed a call in my heart to ancient kauri trees in the Waipoua Forest of New Zealand, to the oldest yakusugi tree in Japan, and to the Hoh Rainforest in Washington state. I know it's my life's work to share my story of reconnection to the forest and to inspire your reconnection.

I'm not a naturalist or a biologist. I'm a designer, writer, and refugee of Silicon Valley tech start-ups. But most of all, I am a human being on a journey of reconnection, here to inspire you to start your own journey through the forest and into the life you may never have dreamed was possible. I'm sharing my journey with you because it is our collective journey. You're not alone. Nature is supporting you, even at times when that's hard to believe. Forest bathing helps us stay grounded and expansive. It keeps us brave and courageous. Anxiety, stress, and fear can get in the way of living to our fullest potential. When we are able to control, minimize, and get rid of ways of being that have become a default setting in modern life, we gain the strength to fulfill our dreams. This is the way forward—it's the path of reconnection for each of us individually and as a whole society.

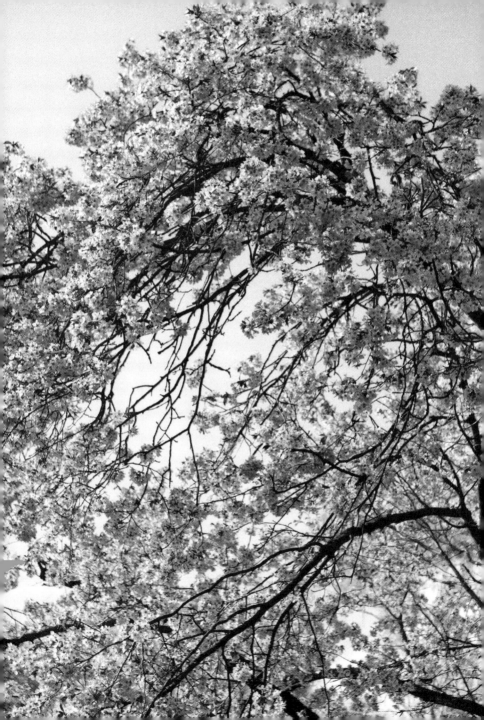

from haiku to
shinrin-yoku

Forest bathing doesn't require a bathing suit, although you might want to wear one because it's great to include some water, such as a waterfall or a dip in a lake, as part of your forest bath. And forest bathing is not an epic trek through Patagonia or a calorie-burning ten-mile run. It's also not led by a park ranger, and no maps are involved. There will be no compasses or hiking poles.

So what exactly is forest bathing? Forest bathing is the practice of intentionally connecting to Nature as a way to heal. Part mindfulness, part child's play, it's a portal into true understanding of yourself and the world around you. Forest bathing is an embodied love note to Mother Earth and an evidence-based intervention to combat the life-threatening diseases that are associated with modern life.

If you've ever taken a walk in the woods à la Henry David Thoreau, you may be aware of the benefits of being outdoors. You breathe easier. The thoughts racing through your head slow down and magically begin to reprioritize themselves—the stuff that doesn't matter begins to fade away. If you're with friends, the conversations may go deeper. You may talk about dreams, intentions, desires, and manifestations. This is your soul talking. It's always talking, but usually we are so stuck in our minds that we don't take the time to really listen.

Being in the forest deliberately activates you. John Muir said, "The clearest way into the Universe is through a forest wilderness."[2] Forest bathing encourages you to hug trees, feel moss, pick up leaves, taste raspberries, and listen to your deep truths. It's about awakening all your senses, tapping into your wildness, and luxuriating among the trees. A forest bath cleanses your soul and allows you to find yourself soaking in nature.

THE HISTORY OF FOREST BATHING

Forest bathing is based on the Japanese term *shinrin-yoku* (森林浴), which was coined by Tomohide Akiyama of the Japanese Ministry of Agriculture, Forestry, and Fisheries in 1982, in part as a way beyond logging to garner value from the forest. In Japanese, the term comprises three kanji characters—the first character is composed of three trees and means "forest," the second character is two trees and refers to the interconnectedness of the forest, and the third character connotes the luxury of being fully engulfed in the abundance that surrounds you.

The essence of forest bathing, however, goes back a lot further than when the term was coined. As evidenced in haiku poems about nature and with the concept of *wabi-sabi*—the beauty of things imperfect, impermanent, and incomplete—much of traditional Japanese culture is based in a deep understanding of and connection to Nature. *Ikebana*, the Japanese art of arranging flowers, for example, dates back to the sixth century; it focuses on a personal and direct relationship with nature. According to one of Japan's most influential modern ikebana practitioners, artist Toshiro Kawase, ikebana helps one realize that "the whole universe is contained within a single flower."[3]

The ancient people of Japan honored sacred spirits that they recognized in nature, manifesting in mountains, rocks, rivers, and trees. Shugendō Buddhist priests, or Yamabushi, are mystics and warriors whose origins go back to at least the eighth century. These hermitic seekers live in the mountains, pursuing spiritual powers gained through asceticism. Their traditional role was to help guide people to one's true nature and to teach discipline and warrior ways. Yamabushi believe that the highest truth exists in nature. Shugendō is a path to help people strip away excess, to understand themselves better through immersion in the power and strength of the natural world. Everything in nature is considered sacred and healing—be it a stone or a river—and practitioners use rituals to honor each of the elements: earth, air, water, and fire.

What religious ascetics have intrinsically known for two thousand years, modern researchers have confirmed with science and data. Japanese forestry administrator Tomohide Akiyama was aware of the pioneering studies of the immune-boosting effects of phytoncides, essential oils exuded by certain trees and plants, when he first proposed forest bathing in 1982. Since then, much research has focused on the stress-busting and mood-enhancing benefits of exposure to phytoncides in nature.

FOREST BATHING AND MODERN LIFE

Humans have evolved in nature; we've spent 99.9 percent of our time in the natural world, and our physiological functions are adapted to it. We're evolved to find relaxation and restoration in nature. Nevertheless, today most Americans spend most of their time indoors, including a lot of time in enclosed vehicles. With the constant stimuli and stresses of modern life, our prefrontal cortexes (the fight-or-flight response center that controls the release of adrenaline) work on overdrive, which means we rarely ever enter rest-and-digest mode. As a result, we have chronically high levels of cortisol in our bloodstreams and are plagued with high blood pressure and other ailments.

We're living in a pivotal moment in human history when the spiritual and the scientific worlds are merging. We're beginning to understand what happens on both a physical and subatomic level as we engage with nature. It's been scientifically shown that spending time immersed in nature reduces stress, lowers heart rate, lowers cortisol levels, decreases inflammation, boosts the immune system, improves mood, increases the ability to focus, jump-starts creativity, increases energy levels, and makes us more generous and compassionate.[4]

In a study spanning visitors to twenty-four forests, Japanese researchers showed that when people strolled through a forested area, their levels of the stress hormone, cortisol, plummeted almost 16 percent more than when they walked in an urban environment.[5] The effects were quickly apparent: within minutes of beginning a walk in the woods, the subjects' blood pressures showed improvement. Results like these led Dr. Qing Li to declare "forest medicine" a new medical science that "could let you know how to be more active, more relaxed, and healthier with reduced stress and reduced risk of lifestyle-related disease and cancer by visiting forests."[6]

In forest therapy programs in Japan, groups are led through immersive nature walks, where they are invited to slow down and rediscover the world around them. They may be invited to smell fragrant leaves or listen to stories of where beloved foods, such as chestnuts, come from. There are breaks for healing bento lunches, meditation, and soaking in the negative ions from nearby waterfalls. These programs may also include nature yoga, woodworking, and soba noodle-making. Such courses are offered across the country, often in small towns accessible by high-speed rail. The Japanese version of forest bathing blurs the line between eco-tourism and nature-focused healing.

With this influx of evidence on the health benefits of being in nature, the practice of forest bathing has begun to spread to other parts of the world, including Korea, the United Kingdom, Canada, and the United States. Forest bathing is the antidote to modern life. This practice may have started in Japan, but it's evolving into a new way of living, which is actually the original way of living—in right relationship with the earth.

For thousands of years, human cultures have had their own versions of forest bathing—of sensorial practices for soaking in the healing powers of the forest. Each culture may have unique practices and rituals, but all are based on the same big secret: Nature is everything. Nature keeps us healthy and can provide the medicine we need. Nature provides us with inspiration and well-being. True innovation and the most advanced technologies originate from the planet. You can read this or hear it a thousand ways, but it's not until you experience this secret that you begin to embody this deep knowing. As you do, maybe you'll begin to see nature connection as I do—a basic human right and prerequisite for true healing.

welcome to the new environmental movement

Forest bathing represents a realignment with the natural world. Indigenous cultures the world over are innately aware that the health of communities depends on the health of the environment. People who live on the land where they and their ancestors grew up are inherently connected to that land. They know how to speak Nature's language and know that we all are connected to the earth. As Native American faith-keeper and indigenous rights advocate Chief Oren Lyons says, "The environment isn't over here. The environment isn't over there. You are the environment." All of us have much to learn from people whose rituals and traditions have preserved a strong connection to the planet.

Since the Industrial Revolution, we have considered ourselves conquerors and manipulators of the natural world: Man versus Nature. This feeling of separation from Nature made it okay to destroy the planet for our benefit. But what we haven't realized is that we are destroying ourselves, too.

As a society, Americans have reached the apex of separation from Nature and are suffering as a result. Chronic illness, including cancer, depression, anxiety, exhaustion, and attention deficit disorders, are widespread and on the rise.[7] These issues affect adults and children alike.[8] With the current status quo, chronic diseases are expected to affect almost half of all Americans by 2025.[9]

The pain and suffering we feel on an individual level is reflected back to us in the state of the planet. Since 1970, the world has witnessed a nearly 60 percent decline in wildlife across land, sea, and freshwater and is heading toward a decline of two-thirds by 2020.[10] As the world population continues to grow, demands for food, water, energy, and infrastructure are putting more pressure on the earth. Massive deforestation, rapidly melting glaciers, coral reef destruction, soil erosion and degradation, extreme weather, and worsening air quality are just a few of the many signs that we've been ravaging Nature at an ever-increasing rate.

Environmental activist and Buddhist scholar Joanna Macy recalls the Tibetan legend of the Shambala warrior. "There comes a time when all life on Earth is in danger," she says. "It is now, when the future of all beings hangs by the frailest of threads, that the kingdom of Shambala emerges."[11] This kingdom is not some place you can go, but rather a knowing in the hearts and minds of Shambala warriors. The warriors are sent to dismantle the dangerous powers-that-be with the weapons of compassion and insight. We all have the potential to be Shambala warriors.

It seems clear that we simply cannot go on doing what we've been doing. But where do we begin? These problems are massive, systemic, and overwhelming.

Sometimes things have to come to a breaking point before they can begin to get better. I believe that all of the calamity and upheaval we are experiencing is heralding a new epoch. At this moment, Earth herself is becoming conscious, enabling humans to awaken to higher values. We have an unprecedented opportunity to create the world we want to live in—one filled with compassion for the whole web of life, and one that we will be proud to gift to our children worldwide.

This shift away from disconnection to the beginning of reconnecting to Nature marks the end of what author Charles Eisenstein refers to as "our journey of Separation" in the essay "The Three Seeds."[12] He writes that the purpose of this journey that started thirty thousand years ago with a tribe called humanity was "to experience the extremes of Separation, to develop the gifts that come in response to it, and to integrate all of that in a new Age of Reunion." We are being called to embark on the journey of reconnection to our personal inner nature and outer nature. It's a rewilding from the inside out and the outside in, as we learn to integrate our hearts and minds and live in harmony with the earth.

If you've been dwelling in despair, it may be helpful to know that several cultures predicted our current difficulties centuries ago: people from Tibet, Latin America, Siberia, and North America prophesied about the future of humankind.

The Andean Quechua Inca, New Mexican Hopi, and Mayan cultures share a prophecy of the eagle from the North and the condor from the South, in which the condor, representing intuitive, nature-connected ways, is close to extinction, while the eagle, symbolizing the dominant forces of industrialized society, reigns supreme. The prophecy foretells of violence and materialism that proceeds a moment of awakening, when the eagle and condor realize that they are capable of more love and awareness and decide to join forces and learn to fly in the sky together again.

The urge we feel to rewild and speak our truth is Mother Earth's own desire. She's done waiting patiently while we selfishly ravage her. She's speaking to us and through us. We're living in an amazing moment of transformation.

As we forest bathe, we begin to understand how to communicate with trees and plants. We gain the ability to interpret a slight breeze or a bird's call. We fall deeply in love with the earth. The more we tap into Mother Nature's rhythms, the more we understand that she wants to help us evolve and live with a higher purpose—all we have to do is learn how to listen. Earth will show us how we can best serve her. As we heal the planet, we heal ourselves.

forest bathing is a way of life

Forest bathing is a modern interpretation of age-old wisdom that does not belong to anyone but actually comes from Earth herself. It's part of the original instructions for how to live in right relations with Nature. Like the three R's of recycling, there are three R's for living on earth: respect, reciprocity, and relationship. As we integrate this way of living into modern life, we will come into alignment. We will restore health to ourselves, our communities, and the planet.

Forest bathing is a journey. What happens during a forest bath is a magnified version of what's happening in your life—it becomes a mirror for what you experience. As you begin to see the beauty in all parts of natural life cycles, you will also begin to see that beauty in your own life.

Forest bathing helps you de-stress and tune out the noise of modern life so you can attune yourself to something much greater and more exciting. This process is less about learning and more about remembering. Truth is, you intuitively know how to forest bathe—the work is to get in touch with your childlike sense of wonder. It's finally coming home after being gone for a long time. It's a way to unleash your inner into your life at the end. You'll learn different rituals and invitations to practice during a forest bath. You'll be able to choose invitations that work for whatever location you're in—even at your desk.

But the real magic happens when you take a walk in the forest. Although you may intellectually understand the forest bathing process, experiencing it physically will change your life. Writing and reading are very mental activities, and forest bathing is meant to get us out of our heads. So if at any time you want to put down this book and take a walk outside, I will be very happy! When you take your journey into your own hands, you become free.

Nature connection is a very personal matter. I've done my best to provide some structure for a practice of forest bathing while giving you space to fill it in with your own experiences and ways that are informed by who you are, what you believe, where you live, and the cultural norms you grew up with. This practice is your birthright, no matter what.

Throughout the book, you will find that the words "Nature," "Earth," and "Universe" are used somewhat interchangeably. I do this because in Western culture, there's no single word to describe the "more-than-human" world. It's my attempt to bring attention to the mystery of existence. Many cultures share an understanding of Earth as a feminine force as well as the planet we call home. Referred to as Gaia, Shakti, Mother Earth, or Pachamama, Earth is definitely feminine. She is us and we are her. If this seems problematic or cosmically strange to you, buckle up for a wild ride!

Forest bathing is a process of *rewilding*, simultaneously the most natural and the hardest thing. It's a stomping out of all our learned wildness. The connection to the natural world is there, even when you're stuck in a cubicle or a traffic jam.

By living in harmony with the natural world, we develop deep spiritual connection to the world that transcends any religious or cultural norms. In Norway, this philosophy of passion for nature is known as *friluftsliv* (pronounced free-loofts-liv), which translates to "open-air living." It connotes a lifestyle based on experiences of freedom of being in nature. When you live in *friluftsliv*, you'll reach a spiritual wholeness that will infuse your life with abundance.

The simple invitations described in this book, such as gathering energy from the sun every morning and giving thanks before you enjoy something that comes from the earth, will strengthen your connection to the earth and begin to shift your perspective. You may find that you detach from things that no longer serve you and connect to people, places, and opportunities that feel natural, even if you can't quite vocalize the reason why.

At cornerstones of the year, such as the equinox or your birthday, and special moments, such as career changes or marriage, you may decide to spend a few days living with the land and opening yourself to guidance from Mother Earth. As you live a life connected to Nature, include her in all your most important ceremonies of your life—you may find that including her deepens their meaning.

Along the way, you may meet people who have answers for your questions and who have questions that you can answer. This is how it is on a journey—the Universe is always supporting you, and sometimes it takes the shape of another human who can show you the way or help you identify a new plant—or a new philosophy. At other times, you get to help others on their way.

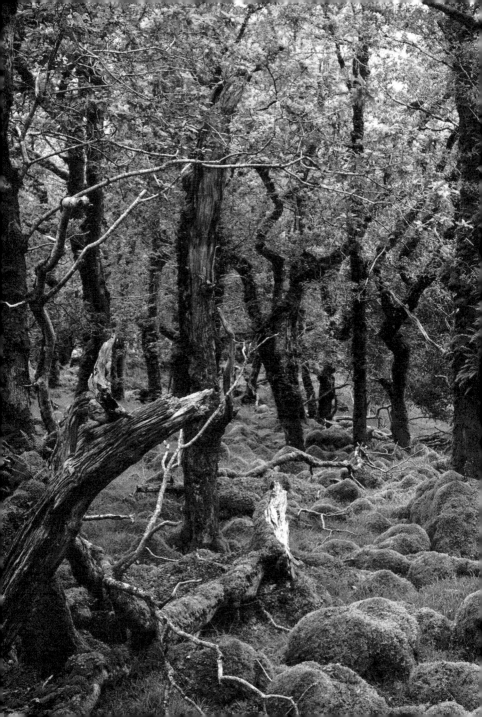

PART 2

HEED THE CALL OF THE FOREST

In every great journey of reconnection with Nature, there comes a time when you accept the call of the forest and consciously cross over from the old world into the new. Bidding adieu to everything you once knew can feel scary, but you bravely do it anyway, because you know there's more out there for you to discover.

Now that you've heard the call, it's time to prepare to enter the forest. Notice what obstacles—real or imagined— come up as you make your way to the threshold of the unknown. Perhaps you feel short on time, car troubles slow you down, you lose your wallet, or something else gets in your way. No matter; look deep inside and trust that you already have everything you need, and keep moving forward toward the forest.

prepare for
the journey

Once you've decided on the time and location of your forest bath or decide to join a group journey into the forest, you've made a commitment to yourself and to Mother Earth. When you decide to forest bathe consciously and with intention, things will start jostling around and your life will begin to come into alignment before you even enter the forest. Changes may be so subtle that you don't realize them, or they could be obvious or drastic.

PREPARE FOR THE INNER JOURNEY

A forest bath is an inner journey to reacquaint us with our own wildness as much as it is an outer journey into the wild. When we connect to Nature, we are actually connecting with ourselves—the part that is so core to our being but at the same time so easily forgotten in the noise, stress, and distractions of modern life.

Prior to your visit, notice your dreams, feelings, fears, and any images that arise. Start a journal, and take some time to note what's swirling around in your life—any serendipities and synchronicities, new people you encounter and advice they may offer. A journal can be more than just writing—you can draw or doodle as well.

Resist the temptation to talk with others about what's coming up for you. Keep it to yourself and cultivate your own sacred container. Take time to meditate or sit in silence and listen to your heart. If you're not in the practice of listening to your heart, you may simply put your hand over it and ask, "How are you, heart?" and wait patiently for an answer. Approach this in a way that feels true to you.

Take a stroll, and find just the right place to be or sit, in a safe place in nature. The transitional times of day are especially potent, during the liminal hours at dawn or dusk. Offer some birdseed, a song, or even a bouquet of flowers to Earth and ponder these questions as you sit:

- Why am I being called to commune with Earth in a deep and meaningful way at this time?
- How can I stay humble and open and grounded to receive the gifts of this experience?

Then, at some point on this walk, take a moment to share your commitment to Earth. For instance, you may state something like,

I commit to the joy of communing with Earth and to come into harmony with all of Nature. Hear me, Earth, I offer myself to you for these purposes.

See what comes for you. Feel Nature hear and support you. Finally, say thank you, share some more offerings, and do whatever else you want to feel complete before returning home.

As you're getting ready for your inner journey, you can prepare for your outer journey. Prepare your body before you go. Eat healthy foods, drink lots of water, and avoid alcohol. Take time to exercise, stretch, and nourish your body.

Gather up comfortable clothing that you don't mind getting dirty. There's no need to get decked out in the latest technical outdoor gear for a forest bath. Quite the contrary—it's easiest to feel connected to Nature when your clothes are made from materials that come directly from the earth. Organic cotton, wool, hemp, and sustainably harvested leather are good options. Look for secondhand or vintage clothes as sustainable options that minimize your environmental impact. Bring layers if you think the weather may change: gather some extra hats and gloves to share and add a raincoat if rain is expected. Ponchos are great because they're loose-fitting and can double as a blanket to spread out for sitting or napping on the forest floor.

Fill a small backpack with the following items:

- A first aid kit (know how to use it)
- A whistle to call out (you won't be going that deep into the forest, but just in case you get disoriented)
- Water bottle and healthy, natural snacks
- A ground cloth to sit or lie on
- A journal and pen for musings and sketches
- Essential oils, such as eucalyptus (awakens the sense of smell and makes a natural bug repellent)
- Sunscreen and lip protection
- Cornmeal or birdseed for offerings

- Moccasins or soft-soled shoes for absorbing negative ions from the earth
- Extra layers and a raincoat
- A bandana
- A hat to protect from sun or cold
- A watch to keep time (so you don't need to look at your phone)
- Musical instruments (such as a rattle, drum, or ukulele)
- A phone in case of emergency

CALL IN PROTECTION

If you haven't spent a lot of time in the forest, you may perceive that it is dangerous and want to stay inside where it's "safer." Such biophobia is a common consequence of never having developed an intimate connection to Nature. If the thought of a snake crossing your path or contacting poison ivy or eating a poisonous berry is just too much to bear, you're not alone. Going into the forest is a way to get over your fears so that you can open up to a lot more possibilities. You can start slowly. You can dip your toes into the forest before you draw a whole bath.

To prepare for whatever may come your way, take a few precautions:

- Before you start out, tell someone where you will be going and about what time to expect you to return. Just as in life, uncertainties and unknowns as well as unforeseen risks and challenges may arise. When you take initiative to protect yourself, you stay safe.
- Pack a first aid kit and know how to use it. Even better, take a wilderness first aid course and learn CPR.
- Do a little research about where you're going, and try to learn about any hazards, such as poison ivy, ticks, or wet and slippery

rocks, ahead of time, so that you can truly relax during your forest bath. Tell your fellow forest bathers about hazards, too. Bringing awareness to these risks will help everyone to relax and enjoy the experience to the fullest. If you're unsure, bring along someone who knows the area and can serve as a guide, to help you let go of any worries.

- Pack extra layers in case the weather changes. It's hard to relax and feel supported by Mother Earth when you're shivering. If you're with a group, pack extras so that you can share if anyone else gets chilly. Being in nature offers infinite benefits and healing, but it is wild and can be unpredictable.

Just as you protect yourself for your outer journey, it's also important to call in protection for your inner, spiritual journey through the forest. Here are some options:

- Bring along small sacred objects that can help connect the spiritual world with the physical world, as well as your inner world with the outer world. This could include crystals or gems such as turquoise, which was traditionally given to people about to embark on a long journey, or amethyst, which protects the wearer while traveling. My most sacred objects are the acorns, seashells, and stones I have found along the way. I keep them in jacket pockets, and a wave of belonging washes over me every time I put my hand in my pocket and find a treasure there.
- Consider bringing personal items that have significance to you, such as a scarf from your grandmother, or a stone or shell you found on the beach during a special day.

- Gather a bundle of respectfully harvested dried herbs, such as sage, to burn before entering the forest. Light it and shake it until the fire is out and only the smoke remains. Always use extreme caution when using fire—this activity is best done well away from any grass or trees, during wet seasons, with much care, and with proper extinguishing methods. Cover your body with the smoke, from head to toe and front to back, to wash away the outside world before entering the sacred forest. Burning herbs is an ancient practice that clears away harmful energy and airborne pathogens. Also, as we burn sage or other herbs, we neutralize the stressful positive ions and release negative ions into the atmosphere, making us feel lighter and freer. Used medicinally around the world, burning herbs and plants also improves lung, skin, and brain function.[1]

When you enter the forest with preparation and good intentions, you become open to infinite possibilities and a more expansive reality.

Cultures from ancient Celtic druids to Native Americans to Asian Buddhists have their own traditions of burning herbs that have been passed down through generations. Somewhere along the way, many of us lost this tradition as we lost our connection to Earth. Now we are relearning it, with the help of the original inhabitants of the land on which we live and indigenous cultures that remain intimately connected to the land. Most important is to do this practice, as well as all spiritual practices, with humility, respect, and reverence for all beings on Earth past, present, and future.

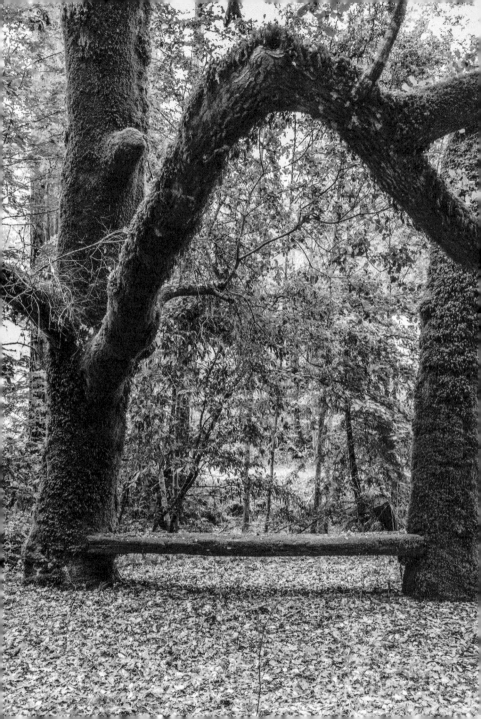

get outside
and find a place

Above all, just get outside. Forest bathing is not a deep wilderness experience. It can really happen anywhere. If you live in or near the woods, just step out your front door. On the other hand, if you live in the concrete jungle, you can benefit from nature by walking in a park or next to a canal. Although it's easiest to feel a sense of awe when you are traipsing through a mossy old-growth forest with thousand-year-old trees that create a thick canopy above you, you can cultivate that same sense of wonder in a city park or while caring for a plant in your home. All it takes is intention and a little practice.

Unlike some other outdoor activities, nothing about forest bathing is meant to be physically extreme. There's no set distance for a forest bath—it can take place under a grove of trees or along a few miles. Here are a few guidelines about what to look for:

- Find a spot that's relatively easy to reach. Perhaps it's down the block. Maybe it's twenty minutes away. Look for moderate and gentle hiking areas without steep inclines that are relatively close to public transportation or parking lots. It's worth exploring places that are farther afield as well, but once you start looking, you'll see that nature is truly all around us—even in the middle of urban areas—so there may be no need to make a big trek. Check to make sure you're allowed to be on the land and that it's not privately owned. If it's private space, get permission before you go.

- Try to find a place that isn't crowded with too many people. If you live in a city, go out early in the morning or during a part of the weekday when less people are around. If you decide to forest bathe in an area with other people, remember that they are part of the forest ecosystem, too. Sometimes people or urban noises may seem like distractions, but they can teach us lessons along the way.

- Look for open spaces. We're accustomed to hiking on trails, but forest bathing is about getting off the well-traveled path. With a more open area or a wider trail, it's easy to follow your whims. If you choose to walk along a trail, just remember that there's nowhere to go, no summit to reach. The journey is the destination.

- Amenities are helpful. Although answering the "call of nature" to pee in the woods is commonplace for anyone who's spent a lot of time in the outdoors, it's okay if you prefer to use a bathroom. Look for a location with a bathroom and water fountain nearby.

- Find a place that inspires you. Maybe you're drawn to old trees or wide-open fields. The more time you spend in a place, the more magic will be revealed to you. Trees are very wise and offer great wisdom, but the desert, the ocean, and the mountains also have a lot to offer. From stones to waterfalls to overgrown fields, everything in nature is sacred. Explore the terrain where you live to find a place that awakens your wild yearnings and evokes a sense of mystery.

- Let the place call to you. Perhaps a particular spot comes up a few times in conversation. Or you open a magazine to a page with a story about it. This is how you know where you're meant to go.

After you've chosen a spot, get the lowdown on the location. Do some research into the geological history that has occurred over the millennia as well as recent human history. See what you can learn about who lived on this land over the past thousand years and into the past few centuries. The more you understand about the place, the more you will feel its significance. No matter where you choose to forest bathe, remember that you are standing on the shoulders of many before you. By considering the context of the land you are visiting, you are better able to envision its past, present, and future.

The more you spend time in your chosen places, the more attuned you will become to their energies. You'll be able to sense and perceive on a deeper level and allow the healing powers of nature to work with you. You'll start to feel alive in ways you never imagined were possible.

In the following sections, you'll learn different rituals and activations to practice during a forest bath. You'll be able to choose activations that work for whatever location you're in—even at your desk!

show up

As soon as you show up to forest bathe, you've already arrived at your destination. There's nothing else you have to do. Sometimes we have the best intentions but let other things get in the way. But those who arrive are meant to be on the journey.

It always happens. People RSVP for a forest bath and say they are excited, but then something comes up—there's an emergency at work, their babysitter cancels, or they get stuck in bad traffic. There will always be obstacles, but those who are ready will still find a way to make it.

This journey toward the light has many twists and turns. The trunks and branches of old trees are gnarled because they have been bending and twisting their entire lives, as they reach up toward the sun. Be sinuous, like a tree; this sinuosity will make your journey most valuable. It's impossible to predict the plot twists and turns you'll encounter along the way.

On this journey toward the light, you will encounter the dark as well; that's only natural. With sunlight comes shadows. We need the dark to have the light. The sun must set so it can rise again. Like the sun, you can also radiate your own light. As you do, you also cast a shadow, and this shadow can make you feel uncomfortable. But there is no need to fear or run away from the shadow. Your shadow invites you to look at truths that you might not want to see. It thrives on being kept in the dark, but it loses its power when you bring it into the light. As Terry Tempest Williams writes in *When Women Were Birds*, "'How is your shadow—your honorable shadow?' This was a customary greeting among friends in Japan, a recognition that what we reject is as important as what we embrace."

When we step into the forest, we bring everything with us. We enter the forest to make peace and let go of all the stress, anxiety, fears, and "shoulds," so that we may get reacquainted with who we really are and what really matters to us. We all have parts of ourselves that feel really polished, and some parts we try to downplay or hide. When we enter the forest, we bring our whole selves—the light and the dark parts. All parts of us are welcome in the forest. Bring the parts that you've finessed, nurtured, and polished. Bring the parts that you try to hide from the world—the parts that you might be ashamed of or embarrassed by. Bring the parts of yourself that don't feel welcome anywhere else. Those are the parts that you can celebrate in the forest.

As you bathe in the forest, you will intuitively learn how to grow and expand your soul and self as well as your relationships in all parts of your life. It may be uncomfortable, and it may even feel like heartbreak, but these growing pains create more room for the breath of life to flow through you. As you learn to trust in the power of the forest, your life will spontaneously shift and expand in ways you never imagined possible.

shake off
the road dust

Our minds carry our emotional stress, but our bodies do, too.
According to the late neuropharmacologist Candace Pert, the "body
is your subconscious mind. Our physical body can be changed by the
emotions we experience."[2] Unprocessed emotions are literally lodged in
our bodies, which can result in tension and disease. The physical body
is always trying to release emotion. If we don't express those emotions,
the energy becomes stuck in our joints, tissues, and organs.

The best way to avoid this buildup of energetic gunk is to release
emotions right away. And a good way to let go of any residual stress
or preoccupations you may be carrying with you, before you enter
the forest, is to shake your body. We may not be able to control all the
stresses of our daily lives, but we can control how we respond to them.
After any stressful situation—from an intense disagreement to a long
drive in traffic—you can shake off anger, stress, sadness, or whatever
else is bothering you.

Maybe you've seen a dog shake its body. All sorts of mammals, from
polar bears to rabbits, shake their bodies to release stress and trauma.

As humans, we forgot that shaking is an easy way to release stress so it doesn't get stuck. As we get in touch with our own wild nature, there's a lot to learn from observing other animals.

Take a big inhale and then exhale out whatever stale energy might be stuck inside. Repeat this a few times. You may want to stick out your tongue and open your eyes as big as you can while exhaling. Then start shaking. Start with your wrists and move all the way up through your arms. Shake out your shoulders and your ankles. Stay in one spot or move around. Go wild.

Once you've shaken off the stress of daily life and cleared out the stale energy inside, you can relax. Relax your forehead, your eyeballs, your jaw, and your shoulders. Move through your whole body, inviting each part to relax. Trying to relax can be difficult, especially when someone else tells you to do it. We spend so much of our day wound up that the tension we feel gives us a false sense of comfort. It's almost like relaxing can feel irresponsible or lazy, but really it's the first step toward liberation.

In the forest, there's no need to try to relax. Just go outside and Nature will work her magic to relax and restore you. Studies show that people feel more relaxed after just fifteen minutes of being in nature. And they report feeling greater vitality, too.[3] Being surrounded by aliveness literally makes us feel more alive.

During the forest bath, you'll be invited to connect to nature in many different ways. It's up to you to answer the calls and try new things. Listen to your body and see what feels right for you at this time.

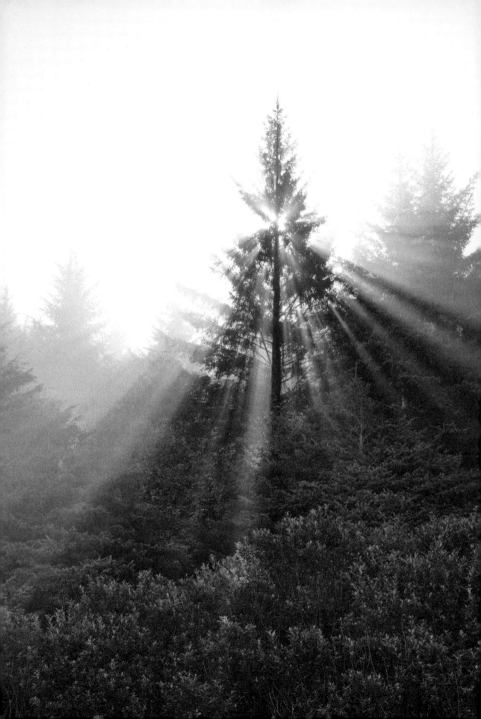

disconnect
to reconnect

A good first step toward attuning yourself to the world around you is to turn off your cell phone. Seriously, stop looking at your phone. Place your phone on airplane mode or turn it off completely; leave it at home or put it away in your backpack. Sometimes jobs and responsibilities don't allow us to disconnect, but for most of us, it's okay to take an hour or two break from our technology tether. You might miss an opportunity for a great selfie, but you will gain a lot more. And when you turn your phone back on, you may notice that you didn't miss anything.

There's so much more to experience in this world beyond the two-dimensional screen. With our smartphones as tethers, we're always tied up. Technology is designed to be addictive.[4] As Jeffrey Hammerbacher, who led the data science team at Facebook before starting his own company, said, "The best minds of my generation are thinking about how to make people click ads."[5] The result is that we're always distracted and look online instead of within for status updates. We're more likely to check in than to check inward. Technology has "connected" us more than ever before, but we are more disconnected from what matters—our inner selves as well as the rhythms and cycles of nature.

When we turn off our phones and leave our screens behind, we're not disconnecting, but rather beginning the process of reconnecting to ourselves and remembering how to inhabit our bodies and surroundings fully. We leave behind the two-dimensional world and reenter the multisensorial, multidimensional world. We will remember how to be human *beings* and not human *doings*. Nature offers us many clues for how to live on this planet.

When you're in the forest, time becomes nonlinear and seems to go at a different pace—slower at times and faster at others. Get lost (or found!) in sacred time. Open yourself to receiving the gift of time. If you're leading a group, assure the other group members that you will keep track of time (and then do it) so they don't have to think about it.

We're not even breathing. Many of us suffer from "screen apnea" or "email apnea"—we stop breathing or breathe shallowly when we look at screens. The apps that we download might be "free," but when we spend hours scrolling on social media, what we're paying with is our attention and health—the most valuable things we have. What we pay attention to determines the quality of our lives.[6] As twentieth-century Spanish philosopher José Ortega y Gassett said, "Tell me to what you pay attention and I will tell you who you are." We owe it to ourselves to look and listen closely to understand the systems and biological technologies that have created the conditions for life for the past four and a half billion years. We must first learn to listen and look to nature to see how we can design technology that is aligned to how the systems of the earth work.

practice presence

Presence is the greatest gift you have to offer. After you turn off your phone and step away from the hustle-bustle of the everyday, you may find that much of the noise does not come from "out there," but rather from within your own mind. This seems like the opposite of peaceful, but awareness of the busy mind is an important step toward liberation. The undisciplined mind is a constant amusement park. It follows thoughts through a hall of mirrors and around the Ferris wheel. It can feel crowded and suffocating. So much of our anxiety, stress, and unease come from our minds dwelling on the past or anticipating the future. We're accustomed to these rides and find ourselves going back to them out of habit, even though they make us feel uncomfortable or fearful. But nature can save us from the cacophony in our minds.

Being in nature supports our being present. Presence occurs when our thinking mind quiets and all of our attention is focused on the world around us. All of a sudden, we can really feel that each present moment will never come again. The now is all there is and if we're not paying attention, we will miss it. Our sense of self, that somewhat artificial barrier we create that makes us separate from nature, disappears and our inner nature merges with outer nature. The beauty we experience can be overwhelming, and we wish that each precious moment could last forever. This numinous feeling feels like love. It suggests the presence of the divine. It transcends shape, form, and function. When we fully experience each moment, life's technicolor and perfect acoustics are magnified. It's not something we achieve, but rather something we surrender into. But it takes practice. And if your mind is anything like mine, it could take a lifetime of practice.

Nature is a great teacher of the timeless now. Watch how a bird, a plant, or a stream exists in the expansive now. Look around and you'll see that today is a gift. The formation of clouds in the sky, the exact weather, and the way the sun's light hits the earth—all of these are unique to right now. Through nature, you connect to your own inner peace and tranquility—beyond the parade of thoughts, that same stillness exists within you. Enjoy being in this state of unity with nature. As you practice presence in nature, you will find that you can bring it to other aspects of your life. Gaze into a loved one's eyes and be completely present with that person. Sit down with your journal without checking your email or your phone. As you learn to cultivate more presence in your life, you will find that you're able to deal with each issue as it comes up in the moment and will feel less and less overwhelmed by what was or what might never be.

set an intention

It's of utmost importance to come to the forest with pure intentions. Everything starts with an intention. It's the foundation of the Universe. Intentions turn into words, which have a way of manifesting into thoughts and actions. Because intention will direct your journey, be clear with your intentions for your forest bath. Do you want to relax? To find clarity with a problem in your life? To bring about peace? To toss seriousness aside and play and be goofy?

Try focusing on intention right now. Take a moment to focus on a desire. How do you want to feel? If nothing bubbles up right away, close your eyes and look inward. So often, we're just trying to get through the day and don't give ourselves the opportunity to consider what we truly desire. When we are able to get clear on what we truly want, we invite the powers of the Universe to collaborate and co-create with us.

Upon my arrival at a Yamabushi's temple in Japan, the priest asked me to state my intention for visiting him. I got nervous and stumbled over my words. I wished I had practiced saying them out loud. He became stern and ordered me to give an offering to En no Gyōja, the founder of Shugendō Buddhism, this mystic-nature connected way of being. He then placed a handful of salt into my hand and instructed me to walk into the river nearby. He sang a prayer while I scrubbed myself clean with salt. He was checking to see the color of the liquid that surrounded me to make sure my intentions were pure. He said that sometimes academics come to visit him and they turn the water milky with their impure intentions.

When you're ready, state your intention out loud, either to yourself or to others. It's important to say it out loud, because our thoughts can be convoluted and complicated. When we voice our intention, we force ourselves to get clear. The more clear and concise our intention, the better. Then let it go—stop thinking about your intention. Don't worry about the details. Although letting go can be the hardest part, it gets easier with practice. Trust that nature will help you work it out at the right time and in the right way.

Just as intentions direct your journey into the forest, you can use them to direct everything in your life. You can take the time to set an intention for each new day, or before a meeting at work or a difficult conversation. When we move through life with intention, we can move through the chaos with determination and conviction. The more accustomed we become to setting intentions, the more connected we become to our true desires and the heartbeats of Earth.

As you become more connected to Nature, you may notice a rhythm to your intentions. Your desires may change with the seasons or cycle with the phases of the moon. It's a powerful practice to set intentions during each new moon. Just as farmers and gardeners know to plant new seeds during the new moon, when the lunar gravity pulls up water and causes seeds to swell and burst, the new moon is a fertile time to plant new seeds in the gardens of our lives.

Aligning your intentions to the pulse of the Universe lets you flow with all of life instead of swimming upstream against it. The ancient Mayan calendar, the Tzolk'in, is a 260-day calendar, with 20 day names grouped into periods of 13 days, or *trecenas*. Each day has a unique tone, and when you connect to it, you harmonize to the rhythm of creation. With this calendar, you can set your intention with the tone of the day. Some days are good for connecting with loved ones, others for communing with nature or setting up your home. It may be that certain 13-day periods are stormy and others are all about personal growth. Instead of the years seeming to slip by linearly, when you attune yourself to the Tzolk'in, life begins to take on a circular rhythm that invites you to grow and expand along with it. Our intentions, like everything else, align with the Universe.

"Intention leads to behaviors which lead to habits which lead to personality development which leads to destiny."

—JACK KORNFIELD

get lost in space

Whenever you feel like the world is crashing down upon you, look up at the sky. Gaze at the moon or at the stars. In Japan, *gekkou yoku*, or moonrise bathing, is a traditional practice of strolling under the full moon to garner its energy and connect to the Universe.

To connect to the cosmos, begin by checking for astral insights for each new moon. Align your forest baths with the lunar cycle. Enjoy the extra energy that accompanies each full moon and take a forest bath to keep you feeling grounded. Stay on the lookout for certain big events, such as an eclipse or Mercury in retrograde. See what happens as the energies shift in the Universe and how they affect your own life. Alan Watts said, "You are the universe experiencing itself."

We can learn a lot about ourselves by studying the Universe. Earth and the cosmos collaborate, just like our brains and our bodies collaborate. But too often, we let our minds rule over us.

Notice right now how you're sitting or standing. Is your head aligned with your spine, or does it protrude forward? With all the time we spending working at computers and looking at our phones, we have a physical tendency to lead with our heads, and this affects how we make decisions and move through life. Although the mind can dominate the rest of the body, the mind seems to be much happier collaborating with the body. Move your head back in space so that it's aligned with your heart and core. Just this tiny motion enables your brain to become more integrated with your body. It opens you up to becoming a channel from the cosmos to the earth.

When we remember that we're part of something so vast, we see that we have plenty of space to exist in. There is comfort in realizing we are so tiny in a Universe that is massive beyond comprehension. There's plenty of room out there, so don't be afraid to take up some space. The Universe doesn't make itself small, so neither should we.

"We are all connected: To each other, biologically. To the earth, chemically. To the rest of the universe, atomically."

—NEIL DEGRASSE TYSON

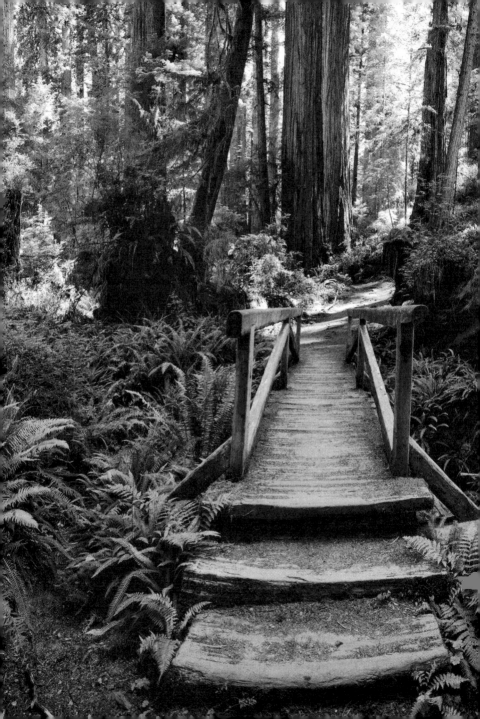

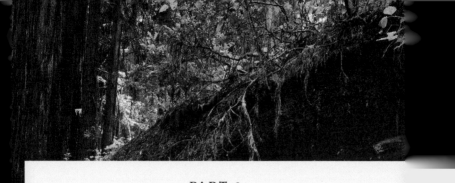

PART 3

CROSS THE THRESHOLD

Draw a line in the ground or lay down some sticks to create a threshold. As you cross the threshold and enter the forest, take a moment to leave behind any ways of being that are no longer serving you.

Living on Earth comes with a set of guidelines, a way of knowing that comes from deep within and that has been safeguarded and kept alive through wisdom-keepers around the globe. If you listen carefully with your whole being, you can still hear these instructions.

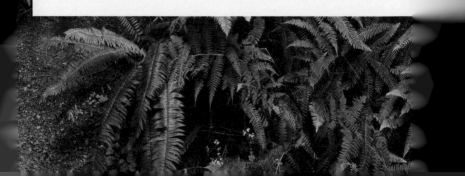

say a prayer
for the forest

Say a prayer for the protection of the forest, for its inhabitants, and for you as well as all others who are journeying into the forest. You are part of a web of all living beings, and their protection is your protection. This is what Zen master Thich Nhat Hanh refers to as *interbeing* in his book *Love Letter to the Earth*. He says, "When we look into our own bodily formation, we see Mother Earth inside us, and so the whole universe is inside us, too. Once we have this insight of interbeing, it is possible to have real communication, real communion, with Earth. This is the highest possible form of prayer."

Look for natural features that mark the entry into the forest. Perhaps two trees serve as a gate, or a big grandmother tree holds energy to mark the spot. Find a place that feels like an entrance, and pause here for a moment to offer a prayer. There's no right or wrong way to say this prayer or lines to memorize. Simply go with what feels true to you at this moment. This isn't part of some established religious practice or a prescribed ritual that might feel uncomfortable. This is from you and sent to the Earth. Speak aloud or sing, give her the offerings of your voice and presence.

- Offer prayers before you enter the forest, and even on days when you're not journeying into the woods. Pray for yourself and your friends and family. The highest magic occurs when you pray beyond yourself; the intention of offering blessings to others will inadvertently heal you, too.
- Start with gratitude. Thank Earth for all the gifts and support she has already bestowed upon you. Acknowledge the love the trees of the forest generously give—they filter our air, help create oxygen and make rain, and they feed the planet—we simply cannot live without them.
- Ask the forest spirits to keep you safe from harm as you enter the world of mystery. They will protect you. Bow to the forest, acknowledging its great power.
- To pray for our own safety and well-being means to pray for the safety and well-being of the forest. Pray for the forests you know, those you've heard about, and those you hope to visit someday. Pray for the forgotten forests and all the creatures who call it home. Pray when you find that your mind has wandered and as you eat, drink, wear, and enjoy anything that is provided by the forest. You may spend your whole day in a state of prayer.

The act of praying is natural and universal. The Buddhist monk in Japan prays differently from the Maori forest guide and the shamanic healer, but they all acknowledge the importance of intimate communication with the Universe.

tread lightly

For most of human existence, we have spent much of our days walking, sitting, and sleeping directly on the ground. We are of the earth like fish are to water and birds are to the sky. In modern life, we've lost our literal connection to the Earth. We sit on chairs and in cars. We live high above the earth in apartment buildings and drive on paved highways. When we do walk outside, we wear shoes with rubber, plastic, or synthetic soles. In forest bathing, however, we can go barefoot or wear footwear that lets us feel the ground beneath our feet, such as moccasins. In Japan, Shugendō Buddhists wear *tabi*, special socks with a separation between the big toe and the other toes, when they go on pilgrimages into the mountains. They believe Earth feels us, so we should feel her.

As you walk and feel the earth below your feet, the way you interact with the world will change. There's something so freeing about taking off your shoes and feeling the soil or grass beneath your toes. It's a little personal act of rebellion against the constraints of society. Try walking this way and notice if it sparks any childhood memories. Many children naturally walk forward on their toes. We are born wild. We are born out of the earth with a deep and natural connection to it. Reconnecting to nature starts with your feet, natural points of connection with the earth.

If your thoughts are running rampant, step out barefoot and notice that your mind starts to quiet and you feel more present in your body. Walk on the Earth as though each step is a prayer. Really visualize Earth as a living body of someone you care deeply about and see that you are massaging, kissing, and caressing as you walk along.

Studies have shown that *earthing*, contacting the earth directly with your feet—in the soil, grass, sand, moss, anything—can help reduce inflammation and chronic pain, reduce stress, improve energy, and improve sleep.[1] Earthing is a cure-all.

The earth is the greatest source of energy available to us. Our planet is like one huge battery that is constantly being recharged from solar radiation and lightning from above as well as from its deep-down molten core. When you walk barefoot, you absorb free electrons into your body, neutralizing and releasing toxic free radicals. The two hundred thousand nerve endings on the sole of each foot pick up the electrons transferred from the earth. Walking barefoot will calm your nervous system and help your body return to an optimal electrical state, from which you're better able to self-regulate and self-heal.

"Walk as if you're kissing the earth with your feet," says Thich Nhat Hanh. In Chinese acupressure, *Yong Quan* (bubbling spring) is the point located just below the ball of the foot, near the center of the sole. This is where the "lips" of your feet kiss the earth. Be mindful of what your feet can handle. It's not always possible to be barefoot or wear moccasins. And no matter what you wear on your feet, there are times during a forest bath when you may want to remove your shoes and walk barefoot.

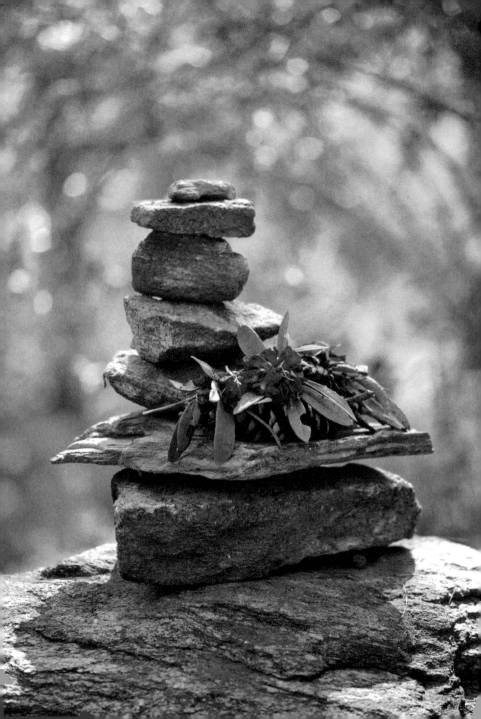

give offerings

Take a moment to make a mental list of everything we get from the earth. Nature provides our homes, food, water, space, oxygen, precious resources, energy, profound beauty—the list is endless. In short, we get *everything* from the earth. You may feel pangs of guilt and grief when you think of all the ways our society has damaged Earth and taken her gifts for granted. Through forest bathing, you can acknowledge those feelings and then let them fuel your generosity instead of feeling anxious or paralyzed.

So what can you give back to Mother Earth? This question can be difficult to answer. At first, this notion of giving back to Earth may seem strange, because most of us are more accustomed to taking from her. We've labeled what we get from the earth "resources" and decided they are ours for the taking.

An offering is a gesture of gratitude and recognition for all the gifts that Earth bestows upon us. As children, we learn how to give and receive. This notion of reciprocity is part of the original instructions for living on this planet and helps restore balance. All the systems in nature are in a dance of giving and receiving. Trees soak in light energy from the sun and create oxygen in exchange. We are part of this dance with Nature.

Earth is totally overexerted from all her giving, and it's time for us to give back so that we can begin to restore all of our relationships. There are endless ways to give offerings. You can create your own prayer bundle by gathering items such as flowers, cookies, spices, and a handwritten thank-you note and wrapping it with paper or cloth to burn in a fire or bury in the ground. You can bury stones or even natural jewelry in a place that's meaningful to you, or toss them into the water. Be sure to only offer natural items that belong on the earth.

Offerings are an important part of bringing health and abundance into our lives and giving thanks for all that Mother Earth gives us. Think of offerings the same way you might bake cookies for a friend or offer flowers to a loved one—a spontaneous and thoughtful act that delights the recipient and nurtures the relationship. Better yet, fill a pouch with organic tobacco leaves or cornmeal to gift during a forest bath. Sprinkle some as you enter the forest, beside a stream, and when you leave or any time you are in awe of the magic of the natural world. A heartfelt song, a dance, a curtsy, and a bow are all worthy offerings to Mother Earth.

As long as you're coming from a place of pure love, there's no right or wrong way to give an offering. It can be as simple or as elaborate as you wish. The most important thing is to be intentional, reverent, and present throughout the process of preparing and making the offering. As we restore harmony in our own lives, we restore harmony to the planet. The more we give, the more we realize how much we are given. Generosity creates abundance. Gratitude begins to grow. The innate notion of reciprocity will again become the way we go about our lives on this planet.

ask permission

As a sign of respect, before picking a flower or tasting a blackberry, ask Earth for permission. (Just like you might ask your roommate if you may borrow her sweater or the waiter if you may order a cup of coffee.) Like the popular kids' game "Mother, may I?" ask, "Mother Earth, may I?" You may feel a knowing in your heart. Oftentimes, just asking makes her happy and she will let you take what you want. But sometimes when you ask, you get a keen sense that you're not meant to take anything, or perhaps you can take only one or two flowers or berries. It's important to respect those boundaries and not take more than your share.

This notion of asking before we take something from nature may seem outlandish in modern times, but the same philosophy exists in many indigenous mythologies. It's part of the original instructions for living on this planet that we seem to have forgotten as a society, but it survives in various forms, including traditional stories and fairy tales.

During a visit to the Waipoua Forest, the largest remaining tract of native forest in New Zealand's Northland and home to the ancient kauri trees, called Tāne Mahuta and Te Matua Ngahere, a local Maori guide told me the story of Rātā the warrior:

Rātā needed to build a *waka* (canoe), so he went into the forest and cut down a very tall tree. It was getting late, so he returned to his village and planned to come back the next day to finish. Meanwhile, the insects, birds, and forest spirits that guard the forest—the *hākuturi*—were very angry that he had cut down the tree without asking permission, so they worked hard to stand it back up. When Rātā returned the next day, he was surprised to find the tree standing again, completely whole. Confused but undeterred, he cut it down again and returned home. Again, the *hākuturi* worked through the night to restore the tree. Rātā returned and cut down the tree a third time. Then he hid in the forest and watched the *hākuturi* as they worked. When he revealed himself and asked them why they did this, they told him that he had insulted Tāne Mahuta, the god of the forest, because he did not ask permission and perform the proper rituals and incantations before cutting the tree. Embarrassed, Rātā asked permission to cut down the tree again, and this time the *hākuturi* happily helped him make the canoe.

Like Rātā, we don't own any of the earth's resources, so we must ask permission before taking anything, be it picking a blackberry or cutting down a tree.

cultivate
tree energy

Trees have intricate root systems that enable them to soak up nutrients and water from the earth and carry it up through their trunks as sap and then into their branches and leaves. A tree's vascular system contracts and expands to pump water up the tree, much like how the heart pumps blood through our bodies. The difference is that a tree's heartbeat is a lot slower than ours, so we don't even notice it. At the same time, trees absorb energy from the sun through photosynthesis. This energy passes through the leaves, down the branches and trunk, and ultimately back into the earth.

Like trees, we are in an inextricable relationship with the earth for the air we breathe, the water we drink, and the food we eat. As American naturalist John Burroughs wrote, "We are rooted to the air through our lungs and to the soil through our stomachs. We are walking trees and floating plants."[2] When we forget this, we become disconnected and ungrounded. We need to reestablish the connection by taking in energy from Earth and the cosmos and releasing energy that's been stuck inside our bodies. Energy does best when it is free to flow.

We can reestablish our roots and connection to the Universe with a simple invitation called *walking tree breaths*, which I learned from author and Shamanic Reiki teacher Llyn Cedar Roberts while visiting the Hoh Rainforest. Try it at any point during a forest bath or whenever you feel disconnected—in the morning before you go to school or work or during a break in your day. Although it's best done while you're outside, if you're stuck indoors, just imagine that you're outside.

1. Take off your shoes and, while standing, rock back and forth and side to side to establish a firm connection to the earth. Imagine that roots are attached to the bottoms of your feet that extend down deep into the ground.
2. Inhale deeply and imagine energy traveling through your feet, up your legs, through your core, and into your heart center.
3. Exhale as you reach your arms to the sky like branches reaching for the light, and let out a "shooo!" sound as you expel energy that's been stuck in your body.
4. On your next inhale, gather energy from the cosmos and bring it into your heart center.
5. Exhale as you fold forward and let out another "shooo!" as you bring your fingertips to the ground. It's okay to bend your knees. Allow your fingertips to soak up the energy from the earth.
6. As you stand, inhale and bring your hands to your heart center in a prayer position. Repeat six to twelve times.

When you feel complete, stand with your eyes closed and your hands together in prayer at your heart center. You may feel both more grounded and expansive and spacious, just like a walking tree.

connect
with a tree

The awareness of energy, or life force, is as old as time. It's known as *qi* in China and *prana* or *shakti* in India. Qigong is the ancient Chinese practice of cultivating and balancing qi, life energy, as a way to stay healthy and uncover our true natures. It's as old as some of the oldest trees on this planet, and practitioners spend lifetimes opening up and attuning themselves to the intricacies of the holistic system.

Among the different techniques is tree qigong. In this practice, you work with a tree to clear energy blockages. You can do this practice with anything from stones to plants, but start with trees. Trees and humans have a special mutually beneficial relationship—always taking in and releasing energy to each other. Trees are usually pretty eager to help out and appreciate the time you spend with them.

1. Pay attention. If you're drawn to a tree, ask its permission to work with it. If you don't experience an enthusiastic "Yes" in reply, thank the tree for expressing itself and find another tree that does want to work with you.

2. When you've found your tree, ask permission to touch its bark with your hands or wrap your arms around it. Take a few deep breaths and focus on radiating loving energy from your heart straight into the tree.

3. Then inhale energy up from the roots of the tree to your heart.

4. Exhale energy from your heart to the tree, and inhale energy from the tree to your heart.

5. Exhale energy from your heart up through the tree's leaves and into the sky.

6. Inhale energy from the cosmos back to your heart.

7. Continue breathing with the tree this way for as long as you'd like.

8. When you or the tree feel complete, thank the tree as you would any other partner and notice if there's an extra zing of energy moving through your body.

You may notice that you stand a bit taller and that your heart opens as the tree's energy helps clear blockages within your body. You might even feel a crack in your spine or notice that you are breathing easier.

greet the sun

The sun powers everything. Without the sun, life on Earth simply would not exist. Sunshine warms us and feels good on our skin. When the body recognizes sunlight, it sends a message to slow melatonin production, a sleep-promoting hormone, and increase serotonin, a neuro transmitter that elevates the mood.[3] As we honor the sun and connect to its energy, we are able to access our own sense of higher knowing.

The Yamabushi monk I met while traveling in Japan taught me a practice to connect to the sun every day. He made sure I memorized each step and instructed me to try the practice for ten days. "Do it each day and be sure not to miss any days," he said, "Then after ten days, consider if it works for you. If not, stop doing it." I've now done this practice every day since learning it, and it works for me. Perhaps it will work for you.

You can do this anywhere, at any point in the day, although in the morning as the sun is rising is the best time. No matter where you are, the sun is always there. Even on cloudy or rainy days, the sun is above the clouds, shining as bright as ever.

1. Facing the sun, stand with your arms outstretched in front of you at ninety degrees, with both palms facing away from you and toward the sun.

2. Bring your thumbs together and place the tips of your four fingers on one hand over the four fingers on the other hand, creating a triangle shape in the space between your hands.
3. Close your eyes and stay still for a moment, feeling the heat of the sun on your palms.
4. Inhale and bring your hands together in prayer position at your heart's center. Feel the energy of the sun warm your heart.
5. On your next inhale, circle your arms out and bring them back in front of you. Make the same triangle shape with your hands.
6. Repeat this sequence three times or until you feel warmth in your heart. On the last time, hold your hands out in front of you in the same way and say this five-part affirmation, out loud or in silence:

Today is _____ (the date)

My name is _____ (your full name)

I am grateful to be born in a human body at this time.

Today I connect to the Universe.

I promise to use my connection as a tool to serve the highest good.

7. Bring your hands back to your heart center and feel the energy radiating from the sun through to your heart. You're connecting the sun's light with the light that shines deep inside you. Stay here for a moment—bask in the light and notice if you get any premonitions.

Just as the sun's energy feeds plants through photosynthesis, it feeds our souls. In the words of thirteenth-century poet Rumi, "Nothing can nourish the soul but light." An important part of connecting to Earth is connecting to the light that powers all life. Just as there are bright, sunny days and other days when you wonder whether the sun will ever shine again, there will be days when your connection to the Universe is strong and days when you will question whether any of it is real. But even in the darkest hours, there is still light.

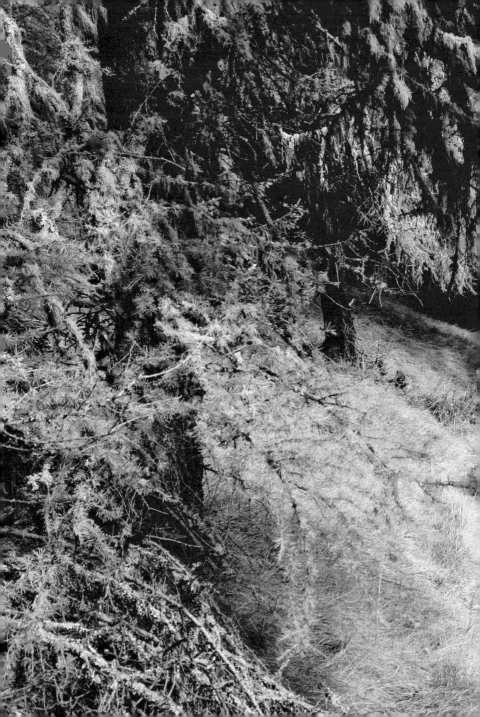

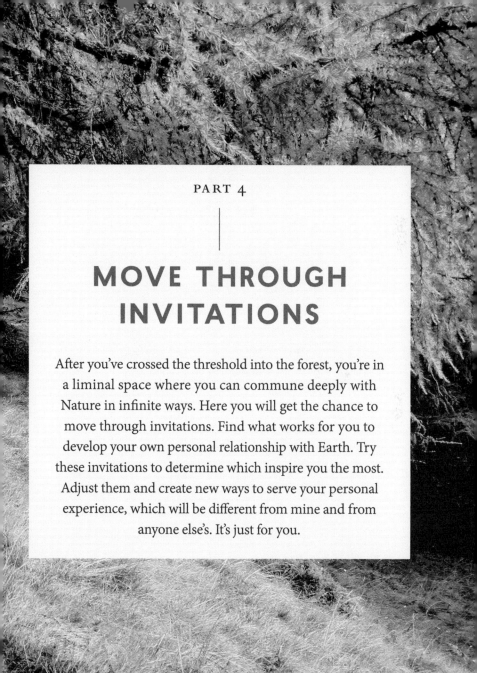

PART 4

MOVE THROUGH INVITATIONS

After you've crossed the threshold into the forest, you're in a liminal space where you can commune deeply with Nature in infinite ways. Here you will get the chance to move through invitations. Find what works for you to develop your own personal relationship with Earth. Try these invitations to determine which inspire you the most. Adjust them and create new ways to serve your personal experience, which will be different from mine and from anyone else's. It's just for you.

walk in silence

Refrain from talking for the first fifteen minutes of your forest bath. This marks your departure from one realm and your entry into another. The absence of talking shifts energy from your head to your heart and body. Silence is a way to show respect for the forest, just as you do when refraining from talking in a temple or church.

While enjoying the silent space, take the time to check in with yourself and notice your surroundings. Imagine that you've just landed on planet Earth and everything is new and exciting. You're part of a team of investigators, and your mission is to report back observations of the planet. You have no idea what those things protruding from the ground are, and you can't help but go over to them and investigate. How are they standing up? What do they do? Are secret messages hidden in the patterns of leaves or in subtle breezes? What do you observe in the colors of the flowers, the unfurling of the ferns, and the fallen leaves and twigs on the ground? What's moving? Invoke the curiosity and playfulness of your inner child.

As thoughts come up, label them "thinking," and then let them flow on. As you walk, you may choose to repeat a mantra such as this one from Llyn Cedar Roberts, "Quiet the mind, open the heart, drop into the body, feel the earth." With each step, imagine emptying a thought into Earth. Repeat this until you're out of thoughts, and then you will hear Earth.

Take a moment during this silence to focus on the empty space between things—that's where the magic lives. In Japan, the concept of negative space is called *ma*—it is the emptiness filled with possibilities and the potential yet to be fulfilled. *Ma* is the quiet time that makes our lives meaningful and the silence between the notes that make the music. What is not there is as important as what is there.

After about fifteen minutes of silence, if you're with a group, find a place to circle up to share observations. Place a talking piece—a symbolic object that you brought from home or picked up along the walk—in the center of the circle. Whoever feels like sharing can hold the talking piece and share what they have been noticing. Only the person holding the piece talks, while others listen with their hearts. Listen with the presence that you've cultivated from walking in silence and clearing your head. When it's your turn to speak, do so succinctly and spontaneously. The wisdom emerges from each person and is held in the center of the circle. This is a place free from judgments, comparisons, and rights and wrongs. When you offer your full attention to another, you are serving them and they are serving you. You may learn something new from other people's observations that will enrich your experience in the forest. And it is healing to be heard when you are speaking from your heart.

After everyone has had a chance to share, you're ready to continue your forest bath. Now you may talk to one another, but keep the conversations in the present—with observations and feelings. There will be time at the end for reflection. If you're in the forest by yourself, continue on, knowing that you are not alone but part of the web of all living beings.

find yourself
in fractals

We've evolved to find relaxation in nature. Unlike the rigidness of city streets and human-made buildings, the orderly chaos of nature relaxes our eyes and minds. Take a look around you. From tree branches to cloud shapes, everything in the natural world exists in the middle ground between order and chaos, both predictable and surprising. It's all perfectly disheveled—arranged just so.

Mathematician Benoit Mandelbrot coined the term "fractal" in 1975 to describe a naturally forming geometric pattern that appears similarly across different-sized scales. Think of the branches that extend from the trunk of a tree. Each branch separates into branchlets, smaller divisions of a main branch, and each branchlet grows ever smaller branchlets toward the tip of the entire branch, where each leaf branches further through veins, lobes, or needles.

Nature doesn't just exist in fractals; it also moves in fractals. In nature, processes create change in fractal ways. From the air, the Grand Canyon displays a fractal pattern created by the Colorado River carving the ground over millions of years, as the river branches into tributaries, which branch into smaller streams, which branch into drainages.

Nothing that's living is fixed or finished; all is constantly emerging. It's the same with our bodies. We are not stagnant beings. Our heart rates are always fluctuating in a fractal process. Laid out on a graph over time, the fluctuations of the heart rate look similar to the fluctuations of a coastline, canyons, or mountain ranges. Our blood vessels mirror the pattern of tree branches or root systems. "This is the grandeur of Nature," said Goethe, "that she is so simple, and that she always repeats her greatest phenomena on a small scale."[1]

Our eyes search for fractal patterns, and when we see fractal structures, a stress-reducing physiological resonance occurs. The fractal stimuli of natural landscapes harmonize with the fractal stimuli of our brains to create feelings of pleasure. This is why staring into a campfire can captivate us for hours, but looking at a lightbulb just isn't very interesting.[2] It also explains why we constantly require updated technological devices such as phones and televisions—we're easily bored by human-made objects, while natural phenomena can entertain us through the ages. When we look off into the natural world, our eyes that once strained to take in a whole city scene can finally relax.

Scan the surroundings for patterns. Keep your focus soft and expand your attention to the periphery. See without looking. Notice what happens when you rest your eyes on a tree or a ripple in a pond. If you're in the middle of the city, try focusing on the nature that grows out of cracks from the sidewalk—the weeds and grass—or focus on indoor plants. Gazing out a window can actually improve your mood.[3] Even looking at photos of nature is relaxing. Not only is looking at nature stress-reducing and restorative, it's good for our eyes.[4] Being in nature protects against literal and figurative myopia.

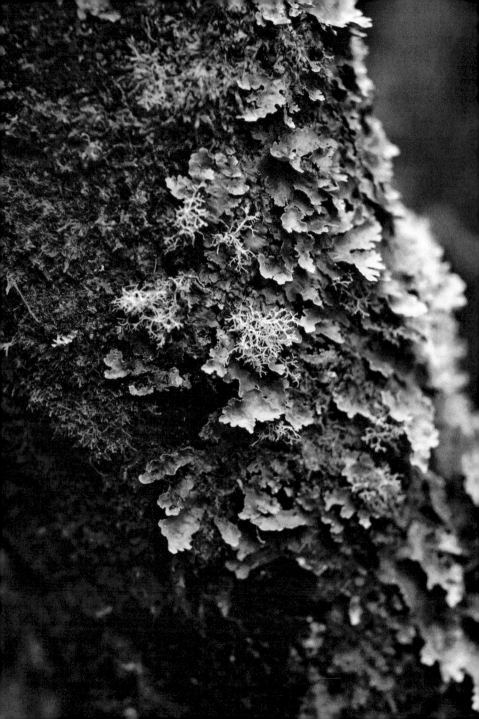

come to your senses

To reinvigorate your senses, practice focusing on them one by one. Focusing on each sense will help you open up to greater perception and awareness. As you meander, invite the forest in with all your senses. Take a moment to isolate each sense; then see how many senses you can engage at once. It's a bit like rubbing your belly in a circle with one hand while trying to pat your head with the other, and it takes practice. Senses are like muscles that we can strengthen by being in the forest. Spend as much time as you'd like right here—sensing opens up your body so that you can fully experience the moment and embody the sentient being that you are.

As the calming forest enables your eyes to relax and you focus on what you hear, smell, taste, and touch, you invite nature to seep in through all of your senses to provide healing. Nature is a healer; you just have to open up to her power and her healing. When all your senses are engaged at once, you are, by definition, fully present. It's a feeling of being alive, and it is absolutely *sensational*.

Nature cinematographer Louie Schwartzberg says, "If you compare light energy to musical scales, it would only be one octave that the naked eye can see, which is right in the middle."[5] In modern life, we rely a lot on our vision, but the benefits of nature are far more than what meets the eye. We take in 80 percent of our information through our eyes, and yet there's so much that we can't see with the naked eye.

SMELL

Dab some essential oil—such as eucalyptus, cedar, or tea tree—onto your wrists and then rub them together, lift your wrists to your nose, and inhale. Repeat this a few times. Essential oils, which are distilled from plant materials, have been shown to reduce the effects of depression, anxiety, and stress, and to lower blood pressure.[6] Essential oils are also a safe and natural way to keep insects and mosquitoes at bay. Each essential oil offers unique benefits. A blend of peppermint, eucalyptus, thyme, and rosemary will help open your nasal passages so that you are better able to take in the scents of the forest. You don't need essential oils to go into the forest, but using them can add a bit of luxury to the forest bathing experience.

Our sense of smell has a powerful effect on our moods. Just thinking about pleasant smells, such as the scent of flowers or the ocean, can evoke feelings of pleasure. The odors of summer air and beeswax have been experimentally shown to evoke happiness. In an experiment from 2008, scientists found that "the natural odors derived from blooming plants increased calmness, alertness, and mood."[7] You can smell your way to bliss. Place your nose next to a tree, plant, or the soil and inhale deeply. Don't try to recognize the aroma; let it dance through your nostrils as you share this connection with Nature. Close your mouth and breathe in the nutrient-rich scents of the earth.

Close your eyes and focus on what you hear. Cup your hands over your ears and listen to the sounds of the birds and insects, and the rustling of the trees. The sounds we hear in nature can relieve stress and restore us.[8, 9] You can hear so much once you quiet your own thoughts and open your ears to listen. Listen to sounds that are nearby and others that are more distant. Some sounds are so constant that we forget to notice them, and other sounds, such as the music that arises from Earth herself, are so subtle that it takes a long time of being in a very quiet place before you hear them at all.

TOUCH

Shift your awareness to touch. If you're standing, notice how your feet feel touching the earth. As you sit, touch the soil, put some in your hand, and notice how it feels. Gather a handful of soil and inspect it. What do you notice? What happens if you rub it into your skin? Get lost in the ancient processes at work in the forest.

Touch is an often overlooked but very important part of forming bonds with one another and with the earth. Sometimes we walk through nature as though we're strolling in an art museum, keeping our hands politely to ourselves. The more we physically touch the earth, the more we open ourselves to her healing powers—and our touch can be healing for the plants as well.[10]

TASTE

Open your mouth, stick out your tongue, and cultivate your sense of taste. We usually associate taste with eating and drinking, but we can also taste the air. Lick a stone. Taste the morning dew. Eat a wild berry. Notice how you merge with nature as you open to taste the world around you.

AND BEYOND

More than two thousand years ago, Greek philosopher Aristotle proposed that humans had five senses. Contemporary neuroscientists, however, have determined that we have a symphony of senses—from twenty-two to thirty-three, in fact.

When we spend our days staring at screens and scrolling with our thumbs, we're not engaging most of our senses and we are not fully present. As we deepen our Nature connection, we reawaken our senses and discover there is a lot more to living than we ever imagined.

As we invite Nature into our lives, we also reclaim our *tree calling sense*—the sense that we have been given a vision, or a knowing, of our path that calls to us from the trees and moves through our bodies before blossoming in our minds.

When you inexplicably but assuredly have to do something, go somewhere, or meet someone, this is your tree calling sense at work. It may work through a strong vision or a dream. The more you learn to trust this sense, the more you will be propelled along your path.

With all of these sensations in your awareness, what do you notice? Do colors look a bit more vibrant? Does everything have an extra sparkle? With all our senses engaged, we experience what mythologist Joseph Campbell calls "the rapture of being alive."

bathe in
the benefits

It takes little effort to reap the benefits of being in nature. In modern life, we visit the doctor when we're sick and get medication to heal some specific ailment. Nature works differently. Instead of healing a specific ailment, connection to Nature increases our general sense of well-being and bolsters our immunity so we're not as susceptible to getting sick.

Research around the benefits of forest bathing has been focused on two components—phytoncides and negative ions. Add soil microbes to the mix to create a perfect solution. Phytoncides are produced to help plants and trees protect themselves from harmful insects and germs; in the process, they help us in similar ways. Negative ions are tiny molecules produced in nature that offer mood-enhancing benefits. When we forest bathe, we breathe in phytoncides, negative ions, and soil bacteria; together, they provide health benefits. These tiny particles work wonders even when we're not aware of them, but forest bathing with the intention of healing magnifies their effects.

Trust that Nature is working her way through you, making you healthier with each breath you take. Being in nature is like being at the most advanced spa in the world. A spa might have a negative ion generator or aromatherapy with some beneficial phytoncides to breathe in, but the natural world offers it all. The best medicine comes from immersing yourself in the whole perfectly designed system of the forest.

PHYTONCIDES

When you take a deep breath in the forest, you may be inhaling up to one hundred different types of phytoncides.[11] The term *phytoncides* was first used by B. P. Tokin around 1930. It is derived from the Greek words *phyto*, meaning "plant," and *cide*, meaning "extermination," and refers to the fact that plants emit special substances to protect themselves from harmful things in the environment. Trees emit phytoncides, basically plant essential oils, to protect themselves; and in the mutually beneficial relationship we have with trees, the phytoncides are beneficial to us as well. We've evolved alongside trees, so what protects them will also protect us.

Alpha-pinene and beta-pinene are two phytoncides found in the forest—released from trees when the temperature rises above 70 degrees Fahrenheit. The higher the temperature, the greater the chemical reaction and the more the fragrance will enter your nose and mouth. Various studies have suggested that inhaling these fragrances lowers blood pressure and increases our sense of comfort and being at ease. Phytoncides also increase our bodies' natural killer (NK) cell activity, which is part of the immune system's way of fighting off cancer. The immune boost from just fifteen minutes in the forest lasts up to thirty days, suggesting that a forest bath once a month is enough to sustain higher levels of immunity.[12]

NEGATIVE IONS

Negative ions are invisible molecules found in the forest, the mountains, and near water, such as oceans and waterfalls. When you visit these places, you absorb the negative ions into your bloodstream, which produces a biochemical reaction that boosts production of serotonin, the neurotransmitter that's responsible for alleviating depression and relieving stress. The negatively ionized air promotes alpha brain waves and increases brain wave amplitude, creating an overall clear and calming effect. In other words, exposure to negative ions leads to good vibes.

SOIL BACTERIA

Trees put down roots into the soil, where an entire community of microorganisms, called the microbiome, supports their growth and nutrient and water uptake. The billions of life-forms that live in the soil transform soil nutrients to make the soil valuable to the trees, and to us. The healing powers of nature are abundant in the forest air and floor. A cure to distress can also be found in a handful of forest soil. Exposure to the soil bacteria *Mycobacterium vaccae* can improve our immune health and emotional health by acting as a natural antidepressant that increases the release and metabolism of serotonin in parts of the brain that control cognitive function.[13] Today we oversterilize everything; as a result, we suffer from an abundance of health issues, from inflammation to allergies. Studies suggest that when we are exposed to soil microbes by playing in the soil, we benefit in unexpected and healthful ways.[14]

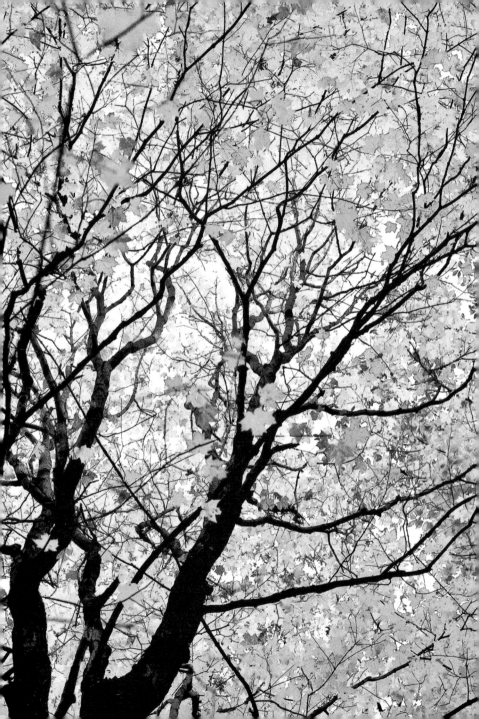

look up

Awe is an emotional state that straddles the boundary of pleasure and fear.[15] It's the sensation of experiencing something that transcends our understanding of the world and has the potential to transform our lives. Awe is eye-opening; it invites us to awaken to new ways of thinking, processing, and understanding. It can help us reconsider our sense of self and our roles in society from a more cosmic perspective, which leads to greater generosity and altruism. You may remember a few times in your life when you've felt a great sense of awe. All of the magic that comes with feeling awe is available to us at any moment. Getting lost in the vast beauty of nature, big and small, has long-lasting, life-altering benefits. When you look up, everything in life starts looking up, too.

John Steinbeck wrote, "The redwoods, once seen, leave a mark or create a vision that stays with you always. . . . From them comes a silence and awe." Research agrees. One study showed that looking up at trees for even one minute could induce feelings of awe, which resulted in increased altruism and feelings of belonging.[16] Such studies show that feeling awe offers several benefits: it inspires creativity, and it lowers cytokines in the body, which reduces the risk of illness. When people experience awe, they report having more time available, meaning they are less stressed, more patient, and more willing to lend a helping hand.[17]

let it go

In nature, certain species of trees go through a process called cladoptosis. They self-prune, shedding branches that are shaded or diseased, as they grow toward the light. As part of the beautiful cycle of all things in nature, the branches that were a drain of resources for the tree decompose to become offerings of mineral-rich detritus to feed the earth. When we let go of what's no longer serving us, we create spaciousness in our lives to nourish what we really want to cultivate.

What you do want to cultivate in your life? What is holding you back from growing toward the light? Whatever it is you want to cultivate and manifest, imagine how you'll feel after you have obtained the things that you deeply desire. Name these feelings.

In the forest, pick up a stick or a fallen leaf and hold it in your hands. Bring into your awareness something about which you feel worried or anxious—something in your own life, something that affects your friends or family, or something that affects the entire planet. It may be as basic as what your next meal will be or something as large and abstract as global warming, income inequality, rising costs of health insurance, the rise of intolerance, or any other significant issues. Your concerns could include a laundry list of anxieties—from repaying student loans to time ticking away on your fertility clock to figuring out the right birthday present for a friend (oops, those are just mine!).

With a big exhale, drop the stick or leaf back onto the ground and release your worried energy into the earth. Don't be concerned about dropping your energetic baggage onto Earth. She can handle it; she recycles energy that's no longer serving you. You may notice that you start to feel better by naming these worries.[18] You may feel a bit lighter and more free. Repeat this process as many times as you need. Many of us think that we need to hold on to all these anxieties and stresses, but actually when we let them go we're able to get beyond the small things that have been unknowingly preoccupying us so that we're able to focus on bigger things. And there's big work to be done.

If you're feeling overwhelmed with life, simply lie down on the earth. Allow the weight of your body to sink into the ground and feel the sense that you are being held. Surrender your whole being. A fern doesn't worry about how it's going to unfurl. Be like the fern and know you are supported. Stay there in Nature's cradle until you're ready to continue. Then continue walking, perhaps with a little more swagger, as you move like you already feel the way you so deeply desire to feel. Look for a portal along the trail—an arched branch or some other natural doorway that you can walk through. When you walk through this portal, you'll be in a new dimension where your dreams are already real.

find
your rhythm

Everything in nature has a rhythm; it's how the planet keeps track of time. Each day has a rhythm. Seasons have a rhythm as do moon cycles, ocean tides, river currents, and weather patterns. Spring is for making new plans and sowing seeds. Summer is for working hard, staying out late, and celebrating. Fall is for harvesting the fruits of your labors and storing them for winter. Winter is a time to slow down and go internal. Each season prepares us for the next. When we align our lives to the flow of nature, we're able to move with grace. Your body is an instrument of the earth, but it might be out of tune. You can tune yourself as you would a guitar to harmonize with all of life.

Every day, the energy in the morning rejuvenates—it's a great time for collecting Earth's qi. Connect to her energy in the early morning during sunrise. As the day progresses, Earth's energy settles and becomes calmer. Around sunset is the time to release the stress of the day and open up to the universal life force. You'll go to sleep relaxed and wake up feeling well-rested and full of vitality.

We operate on a circadian rhythm, the twenty-four-hour cycle of recurring physiological changes that govern our sleep cycles, peak active times, cell regeneration, hormone production, and even hunger. Our daily rhythms change with the seasons, and over the years. These rhythms are governed internally but are susceptible to outside stimuli such as light, temperature, and sound. We are made up of the same minerals and energy as the rest of the natural world, but modern technology has made it easy to fall out of line with our wild rhythm.

Through spending time in the forest, your body and mind settle into a natural rhythm, where your breath, pulse, and steps harmonize together and interplay with the rhythms of the surrounding landscape. Your mind becomes absorbed by the landscape and you are overcome with a deep sense of peace.[19] You feel at home in your body and in your surroundings. This is true comfort. Spending time close to nature—be it camping, canoeing, trekking, or forest bathing—realigns your rhythms to those of the world around you.[20]

Find the rhythm in your footsteps. If you feel energetic, try sprinting or skipping. If you feel tired, take a rest. If you feel hungry, have a snack. Indulge in what your body desires and see what happens. This is the process of attuning yourself to your own wildness. The Greeks had two words for time—*chronos* and *kairos*. *Chronos* refers to minutes and seconds—it's the time displayed on our phone screens. *Kairos* is the opportune moment—it's *right timing*. See what happens when you shift into your own sense of *kairos*. Find your own beat as you move through the forest.

sing with the land

Maybe you're a rock star, or maybe you sing along with the radio. Perhaps you haven't sung in years. Whatever your relationship with your voice, singing to the forest awakens your ancestral memories. Singing is a way to reconnect with your truth, which comes through your soul, into your body, and then merges with the outside world. Earth songs have been passed down orally over generations. Every nature-connected culture and practice has songs that connect them with the earth. There are songs for journeying, songs for healing, songs for celebrating, and songs for remembering. Song-keepers pass on songs full of wisdom and hope. You can learn these songs from others or make up your own.

Listen to the sounds that emanate from the earth. What elements can you differentiate in the orchestra of the land? As you wander, sing a spontaneous prayer song to Earth. Don't get bogged down in carrying a tune, being on pitch, or maintaining a rhythm. Find your own expression. Start by singing what you're doing and then add what you notice and how it makes you feel. Sing your gratitude. There are many ways to sing with nature. Imitate sounds that you hear in the forest. Join in the call-and-response with the wild. Howl at the moon, yell into the waves, explore resonance with rocks, and sigh with the desert. You can bring your own instrument—a rattle, a drum, or a ukulele. Or make an instrument with sticks, pinecones, or shells. Fill a mason jar with popcorn kernels. Keep the beat with your feet.

As you walk through the forest, sing your soul's song for today. The song of today is different from the song of yesterday or tomorrow. It may be long vowel tones or short and quick rhythmic sounds. It may be gentle or angry. Just let it out. You may use words or it could be gibberish. Let the noises come from deep inside. Sound connects the outer environment with your inner one. See what happens when you come across other people while you are singing in the forest.

Add gestures to your music. String a few together into a dance. That's it. There's no need for anything complicated. If you feel stuck, remember that you're offering this dance to Earth and that it's all about play. How might you dance with Nature as if she is leading and you are following? Your work during your forest bath is to let loose and not get hung up. The more you are able to play and release any judgment, the more you invite others to do the same.

get elemental

Once upon a time, humans knew the four elements—earth, water, air, and fire—as guides. Nowadays, we often take these elements for granted, and in doing so we lose our ability to see the world and ourselves in it. But we are all made up of the same basic building blocks.

The four elements interact with every living thing. Luckily, Mother Earth has safeguarded the wisdom of the elements for us, and she offers a living example of how the elements work together. Consider a tree: From the earth, the tree absorbs water and minerals necessary for its growth through its roots. From the sun, it soaks up the fire element. From the air, it pulls in oxygen to breathe through its leaves. Through transpiration, mature trees release hundreds of gallons of water into the air each day through their leaves and needles. Dead, decaying trees release nutrients into the soil. The wind carries seeds to other parts of the forest, where creatures eat them or they lodge in the soil and grow into new trees. For some trees, fire is necessary for regeneration, as the heat releases their seeds from their protective hulls. The elements mix and mingle.

As with trees, we require all the elements to thrive. Each element offers different healing properties, and when we learn the dance of the elements, we can replenish and become the most whole version of ourselves.

EARTH

The planet is more than just soil, and includes wisdom held by great Mother Earth. She gives us shape and holds us. Whenever you feel flighty or anxious, or your ego is driving your actions, stomp your feet on the ground or lie directly on the earth to strengthen your connection to this element. Let everything that feels heavy sink into the earth. Whisper, cry, shout, and share your secrets with her. The more we talk to her and trust in her, the more she will show us her wise ways. Being the densest of the elements, Earth can take all our waste and transform it into life-giving fertilizer. No matter where you are, you can always return home to Nature. You are rooted here.

WATER

About 70 percent of Earth is covered in water, and our bodies are made from 55 to 65 percent water. We all need water to survive, just as Earth needs water to create life. Water is smooth, flowing, and transportable. It seeks equilibrium. Whenever you need to release stress, emotions, or unhealthy attachments, dip into water to let go of whatever you may be consciously or subconsciously holding on to. Take a shower to change your mood and let the water wash away the stress. Play in the rain and let the drops renew you. Make fluid movements with your body. Drink water and contemplate its importance with each sip.

Air is the omnipresent element that is with us from the moment we take our first breaths at birth to our very last breaths as living beings on this planet. Air is versatile and mobile. It's inherently ethereal. Residing in the realm of spirit, air reminds us of all things invisible, inspiring, and uplifting. Air waves provide a clear channel for self-expression and communication. Air holds space in the sky for the birds and butterflies. Find a spot on the top of a hill and feel the wind on your skin. Give thanks to the wind, whether it's a refreshing breeze on a hot day or a whipping force on a freezing cold one.

In the form of breath, air connects our minds and bodies and brings us into the present moment. Taking deep breaths helps us relax and diffuse tension in the body, yet most of us do not use our full lung capacity. Fill up your belly with each inhale and let it go with an exhale. As you fill your lungs with air, you fill your body with life's energy.

FIRE

Fire is the most powerful of all the elements. It is the blazing sun in the sky that powers all of life. It's the lava that flows from volcanoes. It's what burns inside us that inspires us to live out our passions and purpose. Fire brings confidence, courage, and creativity. It represents our yearnings and desires.

You can connect to fire every morning as the sun rises. In the evening, light candles or a fire as the sun is setting. Stare into the flames, looking for shapes and characters and sharing stories. Give offerings or write a message to the Universe with your deepest desires; then throw them in the fire and know that they have been received as the fire devours them. Remember your ancestors, who undoubtedly also sat around a fire, and give thanks to them and for all that they did to make your existence possible.

Build up your inner fire by running sprints or doing jumping jacks and heating up your body from the inside out. Offer yourself encouragement. Meditate and rest. Eat healthy food to nourish the fire in your belly.

ELEMENTAL CONNECTIONS

To connect to all of the elements in the forest, find a comfortable place to lie on the ground (it's best outside, but you can do it inside, too). Close your eyes and visualize your body and soul merging with each element. Imagine that you are being held by a big grandmother tree. Connect to the tree's roots that go deep into the earth. Notice how you feel. Now travel up the trunk of the tree as you are released through the leaves as a breath into the sky. Then spend time in the air, seeing everything from a bird's point of view. Then rain down and land in a river. Flow through the river, eventually reach the ocean. Float on the surface of the ocean until the hot fireball in the sky warms you up so much that you become one with the sun. Feel your whole being heat up. Imagine that you are a ball of light, as others come to you for warmth and inspiration. See that you are dancing and singing with loved ones around the fire. Finally, lean back against the big grandmother tree where you started, and when you're ready, open your eyes.

The more time you spend in nature, the more these elements will naturally balance and keep you feeling calm, cool, and collected. Spend time with each element and muse on its properties and how it makes you feel. Notice how the elements manifest within your being.

converse
with trees

When you talk to trees, you come to an embodied realization that they have much to offer you on your own journey. The trees give you a gentle nudge to move along and grow toward your highest potential. In inviting the tree to talk, you will feel a connection between nature and your own intuition.

As you're strolling through the forest, listen to the trees. Notice whether you're drawn to a particular tree and ask the tree if it is willing to talk to you. As with cultivating tree energy, you'll feel the tree's response in your body. If the answer is no, thank the tree for expressing herself and move on until you find a tree that wants to converse.

Take a moment to inspect the tree: Run your hands along the grooves of her bark. Inspect her roots and crown. Notice whether she is straight or curved, whether she is standing alone or in a group, and whether she is a young and spritely tree or old and wise. Get a sense of whether she is healthy and happy or going through a hard time.

Hold on to the tree and ask her a few questions, as though you're getting to know a new friend. Ask something as simple as, "How are you?" or "What's it like to be a tree?" Ask about her shape and life story:

"Why are you curved?" or "What is your desire?" Often you'll receive an answer right away. Continue the conversation as long as it seems right.

Ask the tree about your own life. Ask for advice or for help with a challenge or an upcoming decision. State your question in a complete sentence. Be clear. Ask the tree for more clarity on the answers she gives you. When the conversation feels complete, thank the tree for holding space, and give her an offering or a heartfelt prayer.

Something happens when you talk to the trees. The answers are seemingly obvious, yet unexpected. They seem to shake you out of a trance. In an essay entitled "Nature," Ralph Waldo Emerson wrote the following: "They nod to me, and I to them. The waving of the boughs in the storm, is new to me and old. It takes me by surprise, and yet is not unknown. Its effect is like that of a higher thought or a better emotion coming over me, when I deemed I was thinking justly or doing right."[21] Trees give us a new perspective that we didn't even know we needed.

I've led hundreds of people, many of them skeptics, through this practice. Some people are eager to share the insights they received from their conversation, and others like to keep it to themselves. Either way is perfect. Sometimes it's fun and affirming to share your story and hear others, but each of us must do what feels true. This is an intimate connection between you and the tree.

If you get anxious about decisions or tend to outsource your decision-making, learning to talk to trees will bring more clarity. You allow the power of Nature into your life when you ask her for help and guidance. You're not expected to go through life alone. The trees will always support you and you can ask them a question at any time.

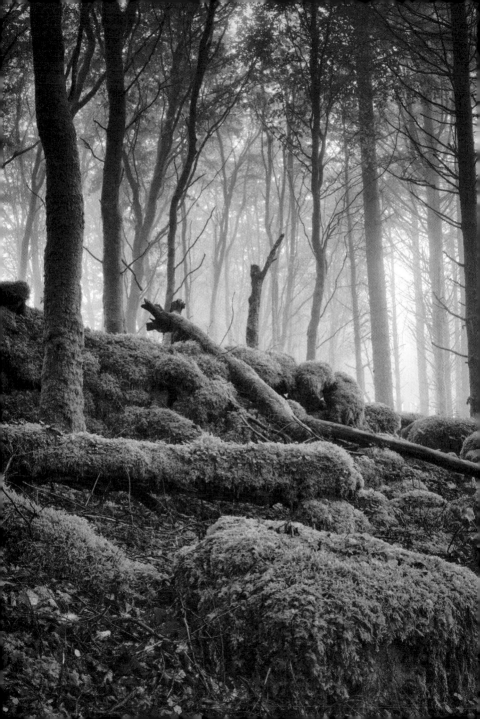

sit in a
sacred spot

Children are naturally drawn to create their own shelters—a secret fort or a treehouse—which encourages their psychological development. If you created similar spots in nature as a child, it helped engender a lifelong love and connection to the earth. Did you have any outdoor hideaways when you were a child where you could go to be by yourself? Remember what that felt like. No matter our age, visiting sacred spots in nature reawakens the child inside and opens us to wonder and awe.

Cultivate a sacred spot where you can spend time. Sit on the ground or on a blanket instead of at a bench or picnic table to create a physical connection to the earth. Your sacred spot is like a vacation home, except you don't come here to get away from it all—you come to be at one with it all. Create a sacred spot to share with others. As your sacred spots are passed on from one nature-seeker to the next, the sacred aura around them grows stronger.

Your sacred space may be in your own yard, in a nearby community garden, or in a corner of a park near your home or work. Perhaps it's near a creek teeming with life, at a lookout on top of a hill, or under a big tree. It's not about finding the "perfect" place but rather a place you can access regularly and easily. Try to stay off a main thoroughfare so you can feel a sense of intimacy with the surrounding landscape. You might have one sacred space at first and then develop more, so that you can regularly visit a few different places. What's most important is that you feel safe and inspired by this sacred place.

Notice whether you're met with any resistance after you find your place. It may seem like there's not enough time in the day, or you may feel antsy when you sit still. Maybe you have trouble focusing when you sit in your sacred spot and become lost in thought. It may feel like you're just sitting there, but much of the work of connecting with nature happens in the stillness. Nature will notice and respond accordingly when you put in the time.

MAKE IT SACRED

To help make a place in nature feel sacred, simply enter it with the reverence and wonder that you would a temple, church, or even a yoga studio. Give the space the offerings of your time and loving energy. Pick up litter, sweep up fallen leaves, and perhaps bring a bouquet of found flowers as you might to brighten up your home. Imagine the boundaries of your space—how far does it extend? Nourish the sacredness through personal prayer and presence. As you support this space, it supports you and becomes a place you can return to, to find inner and outer peace.

Enhance the sense of sacredness by naming your space, even if you don't share the name with anyone else. Choose a name that's descriptive and unique. If a name doesn't come to you, ask the place what it wants to be called.

Time spent in your sacred space can be like grabbing a coffee with Mother Earth. You will get to know each other better and your relationship will deepen. Spend at least twenty minutes just observing. You'll see more and more, as if your eyes are adjusting to the dark. And the more you see, the more questions you will have about all the mysterious processes happening around you. This is good—inquiry is a quick way to personal growth. Visit your space as often as you can, and notice the changes the seasons bring. Watch as the light and colors change over the course of the year. Delight in the growth cycles. Check out what happens on rainy days. See what it's like during sunrise and sunset.

As you observe, imagine you are watching nature TV—an amazing show with a totally unpredictable plot line. Nature is both entertaining and enthralling, always offering us messages—some that you didn't know you needed to hear. You may notice some repeat characters, but there are no reruns or commercials. Bring a journal for noting or sketching what you see, as putting pen to paper forces you to be specific in a way that leads to new discoveries about yourself and the world.

You'll develop your own special relationship with all living beings in your sacred space. Though it's hard to believe until you experience it, forest life will start to adjust to your presence—like Jane Goodall in Gombe Park, Tanzania, where she spent years observing the chimpanzees until they became so accustomed to her presence that they did not run away. Their entire world opened up to her. As you continue to return to this place, you will feel drawn to tend to it, care for it, and protect it. And when you feel that deep communion with your sacred space, you will see all of nature as a sacred space.

eat a snack

Being in nature can help restore your relationship with food. Without all the external noise, you're able to tap into your intuition and remember what, how, and when to eat. Sometimes we eat when we're bored or stressed. We eat in the car or while watching a movie. We eat because it's mealtime and everyone else is eating. We eat to satisfy our taste buds momentarily instead of to nourish our whole self. We eat things that are wrapped in plastic, advertised in commercials, and displayed on a shelf. We're so overwhelmed with messages of what to eat and what not to eat that we've completely lost touch with our own intuitive sense of what can nourish us.

Throughout human history, in times of imminent danger, the sympathetic nervous system that governs our fight-or-flight response has alerted us and kept us safe. When relaxing in nature and our parasympathetic nervous system, sometimes referred to as rest-and-digest, kicks back in, we can relax. With the demands of modern life, many of us don't take time to relax our bodies fully. Going into the forest gives the brain's prefrontal cortex a much-needed break. Soothed by the sights, sounds, aromas, and energy of being in nature, our bodies are better able to digest food in a relaxed state. Not only does food taste better when we eat it outside, but we are better able to metabolize food and process its nutrients. As you eat, take your time to taste each bite fully. With your senses heightened, the smells, tastes, and textures of your food are more vibrant.

FORAGE

As you walk through the forest, notice what's growing there. Foods that come directly from the earth taste more vibrant and alive, and just a few bites seem to satiate. Everything is provided at the exact right time of year that our bodies need it. Leafy greens pop up in time to cleanse our systems in the spring. Fruits blossom in the summer to energize us during these active months. Heartier foods such as acorns fall from trees in autumn to strengthen us through the colder months. Natural foods have evolved uniquely in each region. Indigenous and native traditions that have never lost this knowledge of foraging and eating wild foods can teach us what nature-aligned eating really means. But even if you're not comfortable foraging, you can procure snacks from farmers' markets to ensure that you eat with the seasons.

If you have any knowledge of wild foods, you can incorporate them into the snacks you bring or nibble along the way. You can make healing herbal teas with local nettle leaf in the spring and homemade chocolate that includes wild edible flowers in the summer. As you spend more time in the forest, you will learn what plants and fruits you can eat and when. Nature has her own ways of teaching, often through other people who know the forest well. Ask the plant's permission before taking or eating anything, and wait to hear the response in your body. Take only what you need and always leave some for other beings.

Nature also provides healing foods that sustain us, nourish us, and return us to optimal health. Medicine grows from the earth, where it manifests as roots, barks, leaves, and flowers—sometimes disguised as weeds or invasive species. The forest contains endless herbal and plant-based remedies for everything from soothing sore throats to lessening stress and uplifting the spirit.[22]

ENJOY EATING

Choose foods that come from the earth, including locally grown fruits and vegetables and foods that grow on trees. Before you bite into a local apple, consider its journey up to this moment. An apple started as an idea on a tree that became a bud, which unfolded into a flower that was pollinated by a bee. By allowing its natural cycle to take place, the apple grew with time and patience and finally became the nutritious food you hold in your hands. Without soil, water, sunlight, and bees, the tree would not be able to grow and produce its fruit. It's impossible to remove anything from this natural web. When you bite into the apple, you're in a relationship with all of the energy and resources on this planet. So much complexity and interconnectedness are contained in one simple piece of fruit.

Invest in reusable containers for the snacks you bring to limit the waste you create. When you're ready to eat, find a nice spot to take a break and sit down, and then share a gratitude and bless the food before you eat it. This will ensure that the food tastes better and provides the most nourishment. Every culture has a practice of giving thanks before eating—your practice can be as simple as saying, "Thank you, Mother Earth," or sharing gratitude. It can be a prayer you know or one you make up on the spot.

Digestion is not just what happens after the food enters your belly—it is an entire process that starts when you anticipate taking a bite. Honor the whole process of eating—your outer nature joining your inner nature. Enjoy the beauty of the food you eat. Carefully inspect, touch, smell, and taste each bite. Eat slowly. Give your mouth a break from talking, and let it do some tasting. Let the tastes linger. Keep any conversation present to what you are experiencing in the moment with your food. Notice how you feel with each bite. Notice any resistance that arises as you eat slowly, and just be with those feelings.

There's so much more to eating than scarfing down a sandwich at the office. Although eating is core to being human, we've completely forgotten how to do it properly. Remembering how to eat will help you remember who you are.

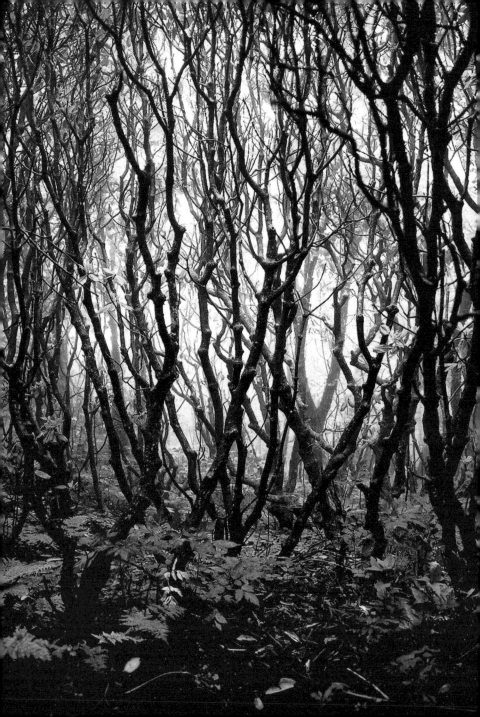

spark
your creativity

To create is to grow. Being creative means inviting the energy of the Universe to flow through you, to become an agent of evolution. It's not that some of us are born with creative gifts and others are not—fact is, we are all born to be creative. But we've been told by our families, our classmates, and ourselves that we aren't creative, or we've compared ourselves to others who have been pursuing their craft for a long time. We've been discouraged from drawing, painting, acting, singing, playing music, writing, or other forms of creativity because we've been told that it's impractical or that we'd never be good enough. Our creative dreams become our wounds, hampering us from growing into our fullest expression.

But this is not the way of Nature. There's no such thing as a bird that can't sing. Each bird sings her own tune. A flower doesn't say, "Oh, I'll never be as beautiful as that other flower," or "There are already so many flowers in bloom, there's no room for me." Each flower shines in her own bright way, offering her own unique expression; there is space for all the flowers. It seems terrifying to overcome a lifetime of negative conditioning, so we hold back our creative forces until, as Anaïs Nin is widely attributed with writing, "And the day came when the risk to remain tight in a bud was more painful than the risk it took to blossom."

When you create, you're joining a powerful planetary force. We are all born out of creation with a natural impulse to create. Earth is a force of creation. It's not that the Universe was formed a long time ago and then suddenly stopped growing—it is continually expanding. And so are we.

In everyday society, there are rules and norms for ways of being. We're expected to be polite, calm, and quiet. Our inner wildness gets squeezed dry. But being with Nature makes us more creative. Nature gives us the opportunity to express ourselves and heal our wounds. She doesn't mind if we scream or stomp or yell at the top of our lungs. Earth can hold all of it. We have to allow these emotions to run through us so that we can clear away all the muck and uncover our true creative voice.

Creativity takes practice. It can feel uncomfortable as you overcome a lifetime of conditioning against creative expression. Just start.

- Channel your inspiration into writing haiku, three-lined Japanese poetry that focuses on nature. In traditional haiku, the first line is five syllables, the second line is seven syllables, and the third line is again five syllables. Don't think about what you are writing, just go with it.
- Sketch in the sand.
- Frame an area with your mind and re-create what you see. Focus on the details—the shapes, textures, and patterns. As you do this, you're capturing a moment in time. Nature is always changing and moving.
- Practice ikebana or your own form of flower arranging.

- Make up a song and sing it or play it on an instrument.
- Gather found natural objects and make a temporary sculpture or a mandala. *Mandala*, the Sanskrit word for "circle," is a visually appealing, balanced structure that you can use as a form of meditation. Creating your own mandala with natural elements is a healing practice that provides insight on your life's journey. Co-create a mandala with others to honor the collective journey. Take turns adding one element at a time, building on what has already been put down.
- Make a gift for someone or offer your art to Mother Earth.
- Choose your preferred medium, such as drawing, painting, or photographing, and bring the supplies you need into the forest.

When you open up to the creative forces that are desperately seeking to move through you, you realize that Mother Earth is the ultimate artist, and as you gain inspiration—literally, breaths of air—from her, you create in her image. Her sounds are the most harmonious. Her landscapes are the most picturesque. Her creations are the most beautiful. Her materials are the most innovative. We as creative beings get to pay homage to the miracles of creation. As Aristotle put it, "Art takes nature as its model."

You are invited and encouraged to play. There are no wrong ways to do this. Nature enables us to tap out of our overextended minds and into our generous hearts. We are drawn to create out of love and respect for the planet. All of Earth is waiting patiently for you to start creating.

take a nap

Far from being a symbol of malaise, as it often is considered these days, napping is perhaps one of the most powerful aspects of forest bathing. So grab a blanket or cloth and find a nice spot to rest on the ground. Close your eyes and imagine that you are a child nestling into your mother's bosom as you curl up. Allow the full weight of your body to sink into Earth and feel her support. You are home. You are held. Relax and soak up the energy. Imagine that you're an electric car getting plugged in for a recharge. If forest bathing is an exercise in the art of "non-efforting," then napping outside is the masterpiece; it's the pinnacle of doing nothing, yet it's filled with so much richness. Stay in this restful position as long as feels comfortable. As you give your presence and time to Nature, she may offer something in return, such as a vision or an intuition, but don't expect to get anything. Just be with the process.

Even a fifteen-minute nap can change the trajectory of your day, and perhaps even your life. Napping reenergizes your mind and body, lifts your mood, and increases your mental alertness, and it forms an important part of the creative process. Speculative fiction writer William Gibson relies on the insights gained from naps: "Naps are essential to my process," he says. "Not dreams, but that state adjacent to sleep, the mind on waking."[23]

Surrealist artist Salvador Dali famously napped in a chair while holding a key. As he began drifting to sleep, he'd drop the key onto a plate, and the noise would startle him awake so he could continue creating. In this way, he was able to enter the hypnagogic hallucinations stage—a liminal place halfway to sleep—and then paint the surreal images he saw.[24]

When we nap, we're able to access a powerful dream state. As we let go of all the to-dos of the day, we open ourselves up to receiving great wisdom. In this liminal sleep state, we do a lot of important visioning. All of us are capable of visioning. Athletes are well-versed in its power. Shamans heal by calling on and embodying forces in nature, such as volcanoes. Children have wild imaginations, mystical friends, and a keen awareness of mystery. But many of us have lost this ability to shape-shift and play with the world.

You need not do anything particular with your visions and daydreams—just notice how they make you feel, and know that you can call on them whenever you need to. Over time, you will begin to cultivate a deep inner vision garden that will be reflected in the outside world. When you find a place that feels like a special nap spot to you—a grove of tall trees or a lush patch of moss—greet it with respect and reverence. Before you sleep, make an offering or give the earth a loving pat.

We often think that dreams are something that happens to us, but it is possible to interact and play with your dreams. Just as you travel into the forest for wisdom and insight, you can close your eyes and travel deep into your subconscious. For example, maybe when you close your eyes you see a butterfly. Follow the butterfly and see where she takes you. You can ask the butterfly a question and wait for her response. You can even become the butterfly and learn what it feels like to have wings. You can do this with anything in nature—animals, trees, waterfalls, or even stones—dancing with the elements and receiving the strength and knowledge that every earthly thing has to offer.

This practice, called the Siberian Mark because of the vision you may receive when you rest your forehead onto the earth, is from Llyn Roberts. I learned it while forest bathing with her in the Hoh Rainforest. She was introduced to it while traveling across the expansive Asian steppe with a Siberian shaman.

- Spread out a blanket (or you can rest directly on the ground).
- Come onto your hands and knees and then relax back so your shins are on the ground and your forehead is resting on the ground. In yoga, this position is called balasana, or child's pose. Your knees may be together or apart, your arms may reach out in front of you or rest beside your body. The most important part is to have your forehead, where your third eye of inner knowing is located, resting on and connected to the Earth. Be aware of any poisonous plants or other potential threats.
- Stay in this restful position as long as feels comfortable. As you give your presence and time to the Earth, she may offer something in return, such as a vision or an intuition, but don't expect to get anything. Just be with the process.

host
a ceremony

Life is made up of special little moments, and if you aren't paying attention, you'll miss them. As in nature, the landscape of life ebbs and flows and holds peaks and valleys. A ceremony brings us into presence and honors the process of living. It gives you the opportunity to step out of the pace of everyday life and into a space of heightened awareness and special meaning. It's the difference, for example, between sticking a tea bag in a mug and drinking it as you walk to work, and holding a tea ceremony in which every move matters—where the tea is from, the vessel it is poured into, how long you brew it, and the way you sip it.

A ceremony is the container, and a ritual is the activity you perform in the container. A ceremony deepens the connection between your outer nature and your inner nature. A forest bath itself is a type of ceremony—it provides a platform for nature-connected rituals. Being in nature heightens our awareness and enables us to honor the gift of life. Specific practices, such as those described in this book or those you create, can become your rituals when you perform them with a certain regularity and reverence for the process.

Humans use rituals to honor different aspects of life. Rituals may be passed down through generations or created anew. They may be rites of passage, celebrations of the season, memorials to honor love and loss, or forms of spiritual or physical healing. Rituals honor the individual as well as the larger community and the earth. Through investigations, psychologists have shown that rituals performed after experiencing a loss, such as the death of a loved one, help alleviate grief, and rituals performed before undergoing intense tasks, such as singing in public, reduce anxiety and boost confidence.[25] Athletes who perform a ritual before competition find that it enhances their abilities, motivates their efforts, and subsequently improves their performance. Rituals even seem to benefit people who do not believe that rituals work!

Nature invites us to perform ceremonies and rituals when we slow down and soak in the moment. Align a ceremony with a new or full moon to harness its energy, or align it with a solstice to celebrate these powerful times of year. A winter solstice ceremony is a meaningful way to acknowledge Earth's energy during this dark time of year when we look deep within ourselves and consider what we want to energize in our own lives. At the summer solstice, we celebrate light and life. During this energetic time, rituals can include lighting candles, dancing, playing music, and celebrating through the night.

The forest bath can be the canvas for a ceremony that you create. Leverage the healing benefits of nature and the elements in a ceremony to improve your health and well-being. With strong intention and a slight shift of perspective, you step across the threshold and into the wild, inviting Nature to participate in your ceremony as witness, teacher, healer, and mirror.

Design your own ceremony. Take a moment to reflect on what you'd like to honor, celebrate, call in, or release. Write down your intention or hold it in your mind. Then perform your ritual, focusing on your intention. You can burn the paper in a fire, release flowers into the ocean, sprinkle wildflower seeds into a field, drink tea, or walk in a circle three times. You can create a ceremony and participate alone or with a community. You may find that performing rituals at certain times of the day, week, and throughout the year and as markers for special moments infuse your life with more meaning, connection, and love.

Traditional ceremonies often include food or libation that brings participants closer to nature. For example, ancient Mayans drank bittersweet cacao, known as the food of the gods and part of a Mayan creation myth, in their ceremonies. Cacao was so revered that it was used as money. An indigenous prophecy from South and Central America predicts that the ancient cacao ceremony will come to prominence again whenever there is a great imbalance between people and nature. Cacao will come forth from the rainforest to help us connect with our hearts, align with nature, and restore harmony on the planet.

Drinking cacao in a ceremony with the forest is a powerful way to honor Nature and can intensify the effects of a forest bath. It doesn't have to be about cacao, though. A variety of plants and trees offer their own types of healing that can be very powerful when used in ceremonies. Bake something with acorn flour to feel connected to oak trees and enjoy the benefits of that protein-rich food from the trees. Drink tea created from flowers or roots. Or create a ceremony around drinking water—every time we take a sip of water, we are in relationship with all of Nature.

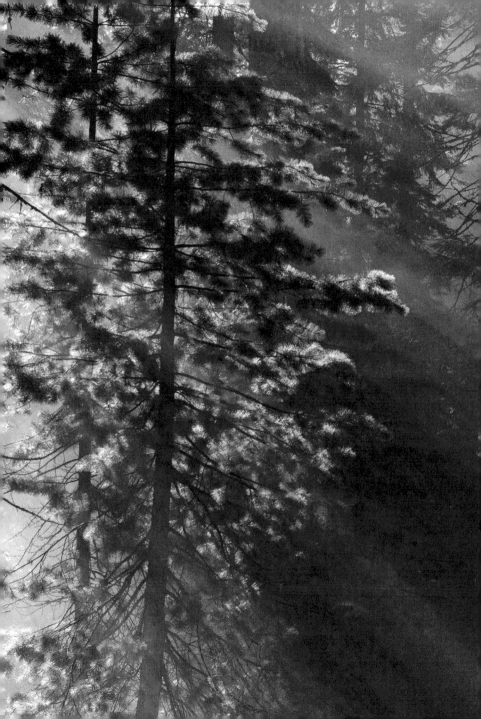

PART 5

FIND YOUR TRUE NATURE

Immerse your entire being in nature and you'll begin to see clearly who you really are and why you are here on the planet at this time. Your discovery of your true nature has the potential to transform your life. Your outer journey into the forest gives way to your inner journey, and you will begin to weave deep wisdom from Mother Earth into your life.

love yourself

Before we can truly love others or Mother Earth, we must first learn to love ourselves. Luckily, spending time in nature leads to greater self-compassion and self-love. As we remember how to love ourselves, we increase our love for Earth. After all, we are all connected in this web of life. We are Nature, so how we treat ourselves is how we treat Earth.

If you often feel compelled to compare yourself to others, when you're in nature, that self-criticism will take a much-needed hike. Many of us know that inner critic all too well. It's that voice in our heads that tells us we're not *enough*—smart enough, attractive enough, thin enough, tall enough, wealthy enough—that we use to make ourselves feel inadequate. We're horrifically hard on ourselves and on our bodies—try as we might, we never seem to be able to conform to a single standard of beauty or success. And more than just being annoying, this inner critic can be quite damaging. It robs us of our peace of mind and emotional well-being and can lead to anxiety, depression, eating disorders, and a whole host of destructive behaviors, from binge-drinking to overconsumption.

When you step into the forest, those feelings of "never enoughness" dissolve into the expansive surroundings. You may wonder whether that critical voice was ever yours to begin with—or just a parrot repeating advertisements and commercials in your head.

As we connect to the web of life, we realize that we are part of something much bigger than ourselves, that there's a lot more to living than obsessing over the size of our jeans. We're able to see that we're not competing with others, but working together, united by our common home on Earth. We can shift our perspective from one of immediate self-interest to something broader and more inclusive. As we move beyond the surface level, we dive deeper into issues of well-being and purposeful living. Nature lifts our spirits and increases self-compassion.

Our bodies enable us to walk on the earth, swim in the ocean, smell flowers, and hear a bird's morning song. As we see our bodies as the vessels from which we experience life on Earth, we open ourselves to feelings of reverence. Where we might have seen flaws, we can see a map of where we have been and where we are going.[1] In a reinforcing loop, the more we love ourselves, the more we love the earth, and the more we love one another. Simply put, loving energy has the power to transform the world. It may sound a bit hippie-dippie until you understand the quantum physics. Positive emotions and operating from a place of love and peace within yourself results in your body emitting different electromagnetic frequencies that can change your experience of reality as well as the experience of those around you.[2]

Ecotherapy is healing and growth nurtured by healthy relationships with the earth. Researchers from the University of Essex found that in a group of people suffering from depression, 90 percent felt a higher level of self-esteem after a walk through a country park, and almost 75 percent felt less depressed.[3] In another survey, the same research team found that 94 percent of people suffering from mental illness believed that contact with nature put them in a better mood.

This is the foundation of ecotherapy—the applied practice of the emerging field of ecopsychology, which was founded by psychologist and deep ecologist Theodore Roszak. At the core of ecopsychology is the understanding that our pain is Earth's pain. So much of the grief, fear, anxiety, and even paralysis that we feel are natural responses to the distresses we all experience, but if we're not aware of why we feel these negative emotions, we get wrapped up in ourselves and are unable to see the bigger picture. In ecotherapy sessions, participants leave the couch and head outside to walk, work in the garden, practice yoga, or play with animals.

So love yourself and the world will change. Thank your body for all that it does for you. Treat your body like the precious vessel that you've been blessed with and accept the responsibility to carry this perfect vessel throughout your life. Infuse a feeling of love into everything you touch. Tell your inner critic to leave once and for all. If not for you, do it for the rest of us. Do it for Mother Earth. Learning to love your whole self is the prerequisite for discovering your true nature and your reason for being alive at this time. Love is a language that all beings have in common. It is the language of the Universe.

follow
your heart

As we strengthen our connections to nature, we strengthen our hearts and begin to move through the world more decisively and intuitively, without constantly seeking advice or comparing ourselves to others. We spend years in school developing cognitive functions but hardly any time developing our hearts. As a result, we take our hearts for granted as mere organs. Sometimes we may notice that our heart starts to beat quickly if we're frightened or that it feels wounded when we feel heartbroken. Otherwise, it just beats. Or so we think.

All living organisms communicate in part via electrical and magnetic signals. In addition to being important for physiological processes, these signals are part of a communication web that is so intricate and complex that it's hard for our linear, rational minds to grasp. Lucky for us, we too can send and receive these signals through one of the most powerful machines on the earth—a beating heart. We've evolved to feel and perceive the world through our hearts and send that information to our brains for further processing and interpreting.

Many cultures and traditions honor the importance of the heart's connection to the earth. The heart chakra, known as *anahata* in Sanskrit, corresponds to the color green and is strengthened by being immersed in the natural world. By unblocking your heart chakra, you open up to greater compassion and trust in the flow of life. In Kabbalah, the tree of life stems from the heart; by opening up your heart, you develop the courage to speak your truth and heal societal wounds.

Most of our current and traditional education focuses on expanding our brain power, but not our heart power. As a result, we feel overwhelmed at the amount of information available. But information is not the same as wisdom. Wisdom comes from deep within us and from deep within the earth. Say, for example, that you are interested in learning about herbalism. You read a lot of books and attend a workshop with an expert. You memorize photos and their descriptions. But how did the first person to study plants learn such information? Before there were books or experts, there were just plants. People spent time communing with, listening to, and learning from plants—what Stephen Harrod Buhner refers to as "direct perception" in his book *The Secret Teachings of Plants*. The world is full of wisdom and teachings, but we must learn to perceive it through our hearts and our senses to access these lessons. With direct perception, there is no middleperson between the truth and your heart.

While walking in the forest, invite your heart to lead you. Say, "Okay, heart, show me the way," and see where it takes you. Perhaps you're drawn to a certain tree, a shaft of warm sunlight, or a pile of stones. Give an offering or a make a gesture. Spend a while just being.

Sit or lie down for a moment. And then, when you're ready, let your heart lead you to another spot. Keep following your heart, bopping around from spot to spot instead of moving linearly along a trail. The more you practice listening to your heart, the clearer its communications, and the more you will tap into a deeper sense of knowing.

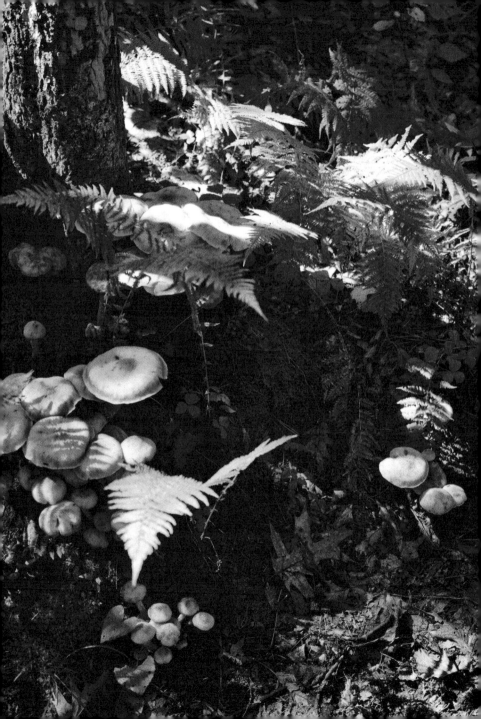

notice signposts
and guideposts

Nature holds wisdom, the deep knowing that points the way. Even when nothing seems to make sense, you can access this ageless wisdom, which will guide you to being your most whole self. You can tap into Mother Nature's higher truths and see for yourself the real meaning behind many wise sayings. There's always something to learn and new tests to pass—nature is the ultimate classroom. It constantly provides signs, symbols, and messages just for you at the exact right time. Nature is always communicating and interacting with you. Just listen.

Nature is also your mirror. What you see and experience in the natural world is often a reflection of what's happening for you internally. Often Nature shows us things about ourselves we couldn't see before. These messages are never hurtful or scary; they tend to be reassuring, often transforming self-criticism and cynicism into something unimaginably beautiful. When you seek wisdom from Nature, you begin a courageous and rewarding journey toward your full potential.

You can practice several techniques for communicating with nature. Use them anywhere at any time, but during a forest bath, when you are already relaxed and aware of the subtle forces at work around you, is the ideal time. The more you slow down and quiet your mind, the more you will experience. What's most important is to be open to listening for and receiving lessons.

SIGNPOSTS

When you're hiking on a trail through the woods, you may see markers or cairns that confirm that you're on the right trail. Sometimes arrows point out the direction. These human-made signposts confirm you're on the right path or point out a new direction to consider. It's important to keep looking for signposts so you don't get lost.

Similarly, Nature offers us signposts, but they can be difficult to notice unless you are paying attention. Nature's signposts confirm that you're exactly where you are meant to be. You may see them over and over again—a type of plant you always seem to spot, a shrub with particularly tasty fruit, or an animal that crosses your path. Every time you see Nature's signposts, she is reminding you that you are in conversation with her and that you're going the right way.

Plants and trees often carry symbolism from nature-connected cultures around the world. A jade plant symbolizes good luck and is a symbol for money throughout Asia. I see it as a sign of abundance. I knew I had found the right cabin to live in to write this book because there was a jade plant in the front yard. To the Celts, oak trees are considered to be storehouses of cosmic wisdom. Whenever I come across an oak tree, I know to pay extra close attention. You can look up the symbolism of different flora, fauna, and animals that you encounter, or assign your own meanings to them. When you locate significant signposts, your surroundings also begin to take on new implications as you step into the world and find yourself in a mysterious, magical storybook.

GUIDEPOSTS

A guidepost points the way—perhaps in the form of a person who tells you which trail to take or a tree that blocks a path you usually travel so you're forced to go a different route. Often, the things that feel like barriers or blockades are actually guides leading us the right way.

To practice finding and following nature's guides, simply tell the Universe you're ready to receive its guidance. Then ask a question. If you feel lost or don't really know the right life path to take, you can ask the Universe for obvious signs to follow. Your guide may be a stranger you encounter in your everyday life or an animal that appears before you in the forest. It might pop up out of the blue and then disappear. Listen to the guide's message. The message may be clear, but other times it seems to make no sense. Not to worry—it's less about what the message means and more about your state of mind as you open up to possibilities.

Consider this—everything in nature is a metaphor. There's a deeper meaning to things in the natural world that we're unaware of in our hectic day-to-day lives. Like creating a language out of hieroglyphics, you will learn to translate the meanings of abstract messages that are offered in a shape in the clouds or obvious messages from a stranger who answers a lingering question you've had for a while.

"Never, no, never, did Nature say one thing and Wisdom another."

—EDMUND BURKE

Maybe you've seen an animal at various times in your life and have felt that it was important: perhaps it's a butterfly that seems to be leading you or a blue jay that appears just as you are pondering a question. It could be as literal as a leaf with white bird poop splattered across it like a Jackson Pollock painting that seems to say, "It happens." The message in this case may be that things happen despite our preferences, but we can choose how we react to them.

When we don't pick up on these subtle messages, they get louder and louder until we can no longer ignore them. Mother Nature wants to get our attention.

The earth offers us endless lessons. Forest bathing teaches us to be patient, loving, adaptable, accepting of change, willing to grow, and so much more. Whatever lesson you receive from Nature is the right lesson at the right time. You may need to practice before you start recognizing signposts, guides, and messages. Have patience and remain open-minded. The more you trust that it is real, the more you will learn.

If you hear or see something three times in a row, pay close attention. I came across three banana slugs while hiking quickly. The third time, when I stopped and watched the banana slug on the trail, I couldn't help but pick it up and move it to the other side of the trail so it wouldn't get squished. It then dawned on me that, yet again, Mother Earth was sending me a message to slow down. I was so impatient that I had to meddle in the life of the banana slug, which was moving at its own divine pace. Needless to say, I'm still working on slowing down and need constant reminders to take my time.

hear what the earth wants to tell you

Beyond presence and love, health and connection, other gifts are waiting for you in the forest—in particular, support for your personal journey, your purpose, and clarity around why you were born on this planet at this time. We enter the forest with our own intentions, and Nature has her intentions for us as well.

As you wander through the forest, know that something—a rock, a leaf, a pinecone, a stick—wants to work with you and through you. You'll feel called to a certain object. You'll see it from the corner of your eye, or it will glisten in a shaft of sunlight. When you find this object, ask, "Are you my *huaca*?" *Huaca* is a Quechuan word for a "sacred object." If it answers yes, ask politely if you may pick it up, and leave an offering such as flower petals or tobacco leaves in its place. If it does not answer, ask it to show you to another object that you are meant to work with.

I learned this powerful practice while in the Hoh Rainforest with Llyn Cedar Roberts, who learned it during her time with shamans in South America. Each time this practice is shared across time and space, it takes on a slightly new meaning. At its very core, it comes from the earth. You can do it alone or lead another on the journey. You will travel through outer nature into your inner nature. The more you practice, the easier it becomes, and reality as you once knew it will bend and break open.

1. Find a *huaca* in the forest.
2. Find a comfortable spot to lie down, and spread out a ground cloth; or lie directly on the earth.
3. Place the *huaca* on your body. You'll naturally feel where it is meant to rest—it could be on your belly, on your forehead, or over your heart.
4. Close your eyes and relax. Take a few deep, grounding breaths and feel the weight of your being release into the earth.
5. Now, in your mind, travel to a place in nature that is special to you. When you reach your place, look around.
6. Notice what you see, hear, touch, and smell. If you're on the beach, you may smell the water and hear the waves crashing on the shore. If you're in a field, you may smell the grass and feel the sun on your face. Perhaps you're by a campfire under a starry sky and you feel the expansiveness of the Universe.
7. Notice who else is there with you. Ask this being if it is your *huaca*. If it answers yes, start a conversation. Ask a question. If it answers no, ask this being to take you to your *huaca*.
8. Look at your *huaca*. What are its features like? Ask it for some advice. Allow it to take you on a journey through the elements. Do you meet other beings? Do you travel to unknown lands?
9. When you feel ready, thank your *huaca* and say good-bye. Come back to that special place where you started. Take a few moments there.

10. Spend a few moments returning to your breath and your surroundings. Slowly open your eyes and return to a seated position.

11. What came up? What messages did you get from your *huaca?* Share your findings and new discoveries from this journey if you feel compelled, or write them in your journal. You may have discovered symbols that will make sense over time or find that as you continue to journey, the messages build on each other. Take some time to reenact the journey in this realm as a way to merge the two worlds together.

As far as the forest *huaca* that you journeyed with—sometimes it wants to stay with you and continue to be a presence in your life, and other times its work is done and you can return it to the earth. You will know if you are meant to carry this object home and add it to an altar or return it to nature. Whichever you choose, thank the *huaca* for its wisdom and support.

Because most of us aren't accustomed to using our imaginal sense, you may find that your critical voice gets in the way. When you're able to suspend your doubts or skepticism, you can journey into another realm, where your altered state of consciousness will bring wisdom and strength from the spirit world that can heal you and propel you along your journey in this world. Journeying is one of the hallmarks of shamanism. It's a tool used for spiritual growth, healing, obtaining information, and working through psychological issues. And everyone can take this journey. It requires no special skills beyond the ability to let go and trust.

discover your own medicine

Everything in nature has its purpose, its reason for being that serves the web of life. Just as different plants emerge from the earth to offer their medicine, we all belong on Earth and have a purpose for being here. In our own ways, we each offer a medicine—a form of healing that is needed at this time. Our work is to discover our own medicine and impart it to the world.

Your unique medicine probably doesn't look like any job that exists. It is a combination of your deepest desires, your talents, and what the earth needs at this time. Your medicine is always in service of something greater than yourself—of people, communities, and Earth.

This idea of medicine is not mine and it's not new age. It's been passed down through wisdom-keepers over generations. In the Lakota tradition of North America, community elders send individuals into the mountains on vision quests. The individuals fast and pray and receive spiritual visions that help inform their roles in the community.[4] In this context, each individual's life calling is considered a gift for the whole community.

In Japan, having a sense of your *ikigai*, your reason for being, is considered the key to living a long and healthy life.[5] Having an *ikigai* is having a purpose that's bigger than you; it gets you out of bed in the morning and keeps you going during challenging times.

Ultimately, your medicine arises from the earth. Every acorn has the potential to become a grand oak tree. The little seed contains all the genetic information necessary to grow tall and strong. It looks like a simple acorn, but it aspires to much more. This concept of realizing potential, known as *entelechy*, suggests that as long as we are able to get to metaphorically fertile soil and receive the nutrients and nourishment that we need, each of us has the ability to grow into the most majestic version of ourselves. An oak tree doesn't reach its full potential alone—it receives a lot of energy in the form of sun and water and information from other trees, and it lives in community with surrounding trees and other forest life. So it is with us, ideally being supported by our families, mentors, and communities. The oak tree surrenders to the mysterious process of growing from an acorn without getting in its own way or looking around to see how other trees are doing it. When we surrender and give up trying to control every part of our journey, we open up to the possibility of what can be.

To discover your medicine, simply ask, "What is the healing I offer?" "How can I best serve the world?" Invite Nature to teach you and work through you. When an opportunity appears, say yes to it. The more you say yes, the more opportunities will appear, and the more clarity you will have about your own medicine.

Like the acorn, your medicine starts as a seed. Chances are, the unique you includes a few different aspects that seem disparate. Perhaps you've felt the need or been told to pursue the more practical side of your being at the expense of developing the creative side. Maybe there are parts of you that you're embarrassed by or that make you feel different, and you wish they'd go away. These parts are especially important and deserve to be revered. Trust that you are whole, that all your pieces fit together, and that the right time to discover your medicine is now.

You may have some notion of your own medicine or you may not have a clue. Oftentimes, the medicine that we offer is the medicine that we need the most. Our hardships become our opportunities. The wisdom, strength, and courage we receive from healing ourselves become our greatest offerings to the world. We have to commit to healing our own wounds before we are able to offer our medicine to others.

You may not have the words to describe your medicine—it isn't something that comes from your mind, but rather from a deeper place within. Let go of having to know. Your medicine may change over time as you grow and evolve. Just know that you offer a form of healing—it could be through art, music, writing, teaching, speaking, guiding, or so many other ways—and every time you offer it, you are providing a service. As human beings on this planet at this time, our highest form of being is in service. We are here to restore the earth.

When you step into the forest, you begin your journey down your own wild path, which doesn't look like anyone else's path. Nature begins healing you as you start to feel more grounded, relaxed, present, healthy, and inspired. You will know that you belong on this earth, perhaps after many years of feeling like no matter how hard you try, you can't quite fit into the boxes, roles, and groups that have been forced upon you.

You may have come to the forest for some relaxation so that you can continue your normal life. But the more times you return and the deeper you go into the forest, the deeper you go into your own wild soul. You will begin to meet others who are also on their own paths to discovery—they may offer you support and you may also support them. You may meet others who offer similar medicine to yours, but trust that yours is different and is uniquely needed, too.

Use the practices and invitations in this book as you start to find your own medicine. Offer up the wisdom you receive. Share and teach before you feel completely ready—by sharing your own discoveries, you lead others to their own healing and their own medicine. It's okay to make mistakes. The more you practice, the more you'll know when you are sharing your truth because it is not something you've memorized from a textbook. Truth comes from your life experience; it's raw and real to you, and you may feel vulnerable sharing it. It might feel scary to put yourself out there, but do it anyway, because you're beyond catering to your ego—you are connected to Nature now and committed to serving the highest good no matter what it takes.

"Before we awaken, our joy is to use the things of this earth; after the grace of awakening, our joy is to serve the things of this earth. With the growth of wisdom, our life becomes more and more a creative act, an act of service."

—JACK KORNFIELD, *After the Ecstasy, the Laundry*

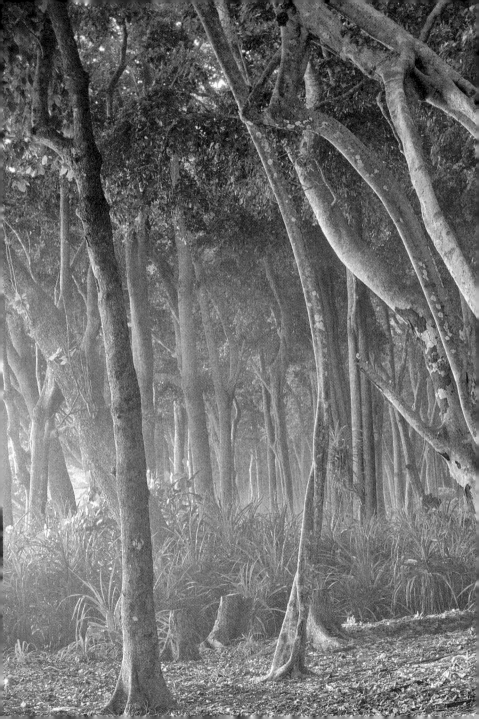

PART 6

RETURN WITH YOUR ELIXIR

How you end your forest bath is just as important as how you begin. You've traveled to another realm, so take some time to close the portal and cross back over the threshold consciously and graciously. Here are some guidelines that will help you step out of the forest physically while bringing it with you in your heart.

The intention is not to separate forest bathing from regular life; it's not to run off into the wilderness to get away. Instead, the intention is to integrate the wisdom of the forest with your everyday life and create a new way of being. This process takes time. Be gentle with yourself and others, and you'll notice a ripple effect: as more and more people connect to Nature and share what they learn with others, large-scale reconnection and transformation will no longer be a far-fetched dream.

thank the forest

You expressed gratitude to the forest on the way in and gave offerings throughout your journey. Thank the forest on your way out, too. Thank her for keeping you safe, for sharing her magic and healing powers with you, for the inspiration and wisdom you received, and the space she held for you to discover yourself. Then thank the forest some more. Thank her for her patience, wisdom, and infinite, ever-evolving beauty.

Thank the forest for things that you wish *you* were thanked for more often—for showing up, enduring hardship, being resilient, and standing strong. Be specific. Thank the soil, air, birds, insects, plants, and whatever else comes to mind. Thank the forest, park, or backyard you visited, and thank forests near and far. Let your gratitude overflow from within you, and you can't help but to share it with others. Your list may go on and on. Gratitude is a truly renewable resource.

When we complain about everything that is going wrong, we create exhaust—the polluting energy that exhausts us. We eventually run out of steam and things to say, or we end up in an anxious panic. But as we give thanks to the forest, we create a joyful energy that uplifts us, others around us, and Earth herself.

Practice this way of gratitude throughout life. When you notice you start to get anxious or stressed, start listing things that you are grateful for. During challenging times when you're walking up a hill that seems to go on forever or just sitting in bad traffic, list everything that you are grateful for. When you can't sleep at night, start counting blessings, like sheep.

Practice gratitude every day, and you may find that the sun shines brighter, colors are more vivid, smells are more divine, and the world is more full of joy. Gratitude improves well-being. People who are grateful—who keep gratitude journals, go out of their way to thank people, or acknowledge the abundance in their lives—experience fewer aches and pains and feel healthier. They also experience more sensitivity and empathy, have higher self-esteem, and literally sleep more soundly.[1]

The benefits of expressing gratitude are very similar to the benefits of spending time with Nature, and this is not just happenstance—the two are intertwined. Being in the wild and expressing gratitude will each place you on the highway to increased personal well-being. Bringing the two together in a practice of extending gratitude toward Nature and being grateful while in nature deepens the benefits of both, like being on a well-being rocket ship. Getting out of our own heads and noticing the nature around us makes gratitude our natural state of being.

take time
to reflect

By now you've received your elixir from the forest and you're heading back across the threshold to where you began. After you leave the forest, before you turn on your phone or get into your car, take some time to reflect. You may have experienced a huge breakthrough, or something more subtle may have occurred. Sometimes it takes a while for the effects of forest bathing to reveal themselves. Reflection is the key to embodying the wisdom you receive. It is the intentional attempt to synthesize, abstract, and articulate important lessons.[2]

If you're alone, take a few minutes to write down any insights or messages you received during your time in the forest. Sit on a rock or a log and ask, "Who am I? Where am I coming from? And where am I going?" Nature shows us a reflection of ourselves: What do you see? Sometimes the waters are muddy and you must be patient as they clear. At other times you can see exactly who you are and what your next actions must be. In this space of heightened awareness, take note of what you'd like to nurture in your life and what you'd like to release. Take advantage of a few precious moments to consider how you want to show up in the world.

If you're with a group, find an open area to form a council circle. Use a talking piece and give each person a chance to share their story and reflection. Their stories will inspire and amaze you. Each person will have a different story, and each person's findings and discoveries will deepen your own experience. They will notice things that you missed, and they may have lessons for you, just as you do for them. Honor what each person shares by acknowledging and mirroring it back to them. Leave plenty of spacious silence between each speaker. Thank one another for sharing what is true at this moment. Sharing in this way may help make sense of something you experienced. Perhaps you have a question about an animal, tree, or plant you saw in the forest. If someone asks a question, ask it back to them instead of answering it: "Well, what do you think?" If you don't have an answer, simply say, "I don't know."

Today we have the internet at our fingertips, and we've become obsessed with needing immediate answers. But often there's more value in embracing the mystery. Answers can sometimes lead us astray. We say, "Oh, yes, that is a bay tree," and we think we know all about the tree so we stop being curious about it. But there's so much that we don't understand about every living thing. The goal is not to know everything, but to be open to the mystery of it all. Through reflecting on your own or within a group, you can integrate the lessons from the forest into your life.

"We do not learn from experience . . . we learn from reflecting on experience."

–JOHN DEWEY

keep the
connection alive

"Before enlightenment, chop wood, carry water. After enlightenment, chop wood, carry water." In this traditional Zen saying, the idea is that how you do *anything* is how you do *everything*. You're not always going to be in the forest, but the real work is to bring that reverence, peace, and awareness that you cultivated in the forest into all aspects of your daily life. In a two-hour forest bath, you may have experiences that enable you to connect deeper to the mystery of life. A single experience is enough to transform everything. Once you've communed with Nature, you can recall that interconnectedness at any moment.

Even brushing your teeth is an opportunity to thank Earth for the water. When you take a sip of water, you are in a relationship with every element. Astrophysicist Neil deGrasse Tyson said, "There are more molecules of water in a cup of water than cups of water in all the world's oceans. This means that some molecules in every cup of water you drink passed through the kidneys of Genghis Khan, Napoleon, Abe Lincoln, or any other historical person of your choosing."[3]

Pray to the water that comes out of the tap the same way you might pray to a stream. As Navajo and Lakota activist Pat McCabe, known as Woman Stands Shining, explains, "It's good for you to pray into the water because it actually intensifies your prayer. So literally, you know that water evaporates and can travel through the clouds. Your intentions and your words travel through the clouds and they can go anywhere they want to go."[4] These same activities—brushing your teeth or drinking water—that you've done every day of your life will feel different with heightened awareness from forest bathing.

Bring Nature into your everyday life. Design a daily routine based on the practices in this book to stay deeply connected to Nature, even on days when you don't have hours to spend wandering through the forest. Set an intention for the day every morning when you open your eyes, before you look at your phone. Breathe with the trees and connect to the sun as you start your day. Pour out a little bit of your morning tea as an offering to Mother Earth. Say thanks in gratitude before taking your first bite of breakfast.

Place objects you've collected during forest baths—shells, pinecones, stones, and feathers—at your desk, in your car, and around your home to remind you of being in nature. Glancing at them or holding them is like taking a ten-second forest bath.

If you start to feel anxious, find a connection to the Universe. Dab some woody essential oil on your wrist and take a few big inhales and exhales, light a candle and watch the flame, water a plant, or look at some pictures of nature. Take a walk and focus on counting your breaths, or sing a song to the earth. Soak in a hot bath while listening to relaxing sounds. Or simply place your feet on the floor while you're sitting inside and imagine your connection to Mother Earth. It doesn't take much—just a dash of Nature and a small shift in perspective can transform a situation.

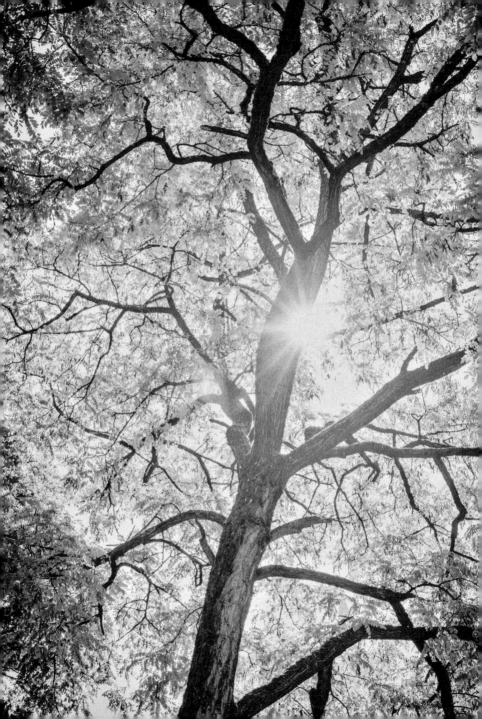

share nutrients

When we understand what happens in the forest ecosystem, we more fully understand our own roles in the web of life. Nature is full of examples of sustainable systems that we can emulate and apply to our daily lives. One of the most basic tenets we can learn from the forest is how to share and support one another.

Trees are connected below the ground by mycorrhizal fungi—the "wood wide web." Mycorrhizal fungi live symbiotically with the roots of the trees; they depend on each other to survive. The trees provide the fungi with photosynthate—the sugar compounds that feed the fungi—and the fungi extend the trees' root systems to help the trees access minerals from the soil. The fungi also connect the root systems of groups of trees, which enables them to share information and nutrients across this underground web. This system is pervasive—around 90 percent of land plants are connected to each other in this way.[5]

The relationship between trees and mycorrhizae strengthens the immunity of the forest and helps support the health of the entire ecosystem. Older, more established trees pass along nutrients to young seedlings so that they stand a chance of growing stronger. The oldest, largest trees are hubs that send out food and warnings in all directions.

Trees will even share nutrients across different species—they know that the strength of the forest depends on the strength of the weakest tree. For example, in winter when aspens are weaker, nearby conifers, which fare better in winter, pass along food to help keep the aspens healthy. If one tree is attacked by insects, it distributes chemicals through the underground fungal network to warn other trees of a possible attack and enables them to defend themselves by changing the chemical makeup of their leaves.[6]

As the ultimate sacrifice, a dying tree will release its no longer needed resources into the network so other trees can benefit from them. The end of life for a tree is really just the beginning of life for something else. As it slowly decomposes, the tree transforms into nutrient-rich compost that can continue to support the cycle.

And so it is with us. We can transform the end of one thing into the beginning of something else. And we use our powerful networks to support one another. We can stay connected to the web of life even when we're not in the forest by sharing nutrients, resources, and information just like trees. In this way, we cooperate and live in partnership. As you extend love and support to others, you're acting as a force of the Universe. Share the peace and wisdom you receive from the forest, or share your time and energy with others. Plant trees, volunteer, talk to your neighbors—there are so many ways to share the nutrients you receive. Like the symbiotic relationship between fungi and trees, the act of giving and sharing is mutually beneficial.

designate
a prayer tree

Designate a tree in your neighborhood as a prayer tree, as a way to integrate the wisdom of the forest into your everyday life. A prayer tree is a beacon of connection to the community as well as to the earth below and the sky above. The tree could be on your street, at your school, or near your office. It could be tucked away or highly visible. It might be an old grandmother tree or a younger tree.

Be clear with your intention in designating this tree as a prayer tree. Share your heartfelt gratitude with the tree, and sit below her as you express your wishes for your self, your community, and all of life. As you bless the tree in a way that feels true to you, know that the tree is a living being that receives your prayer and right away begins to work with the Universe to manifest your most heartfelt desires.

The act of designating prayer trees, sometimes called peace trees or wishing trees, is rooted in traditions around the world:[7]

- At the ruins of an ancient temple in Göbekli Tepe in southeastern Turkey, people visit the wishing tree, an old mulberry tree that grows at the highest point on the site. Believers make offerings to the sacred tree to gain fulfillment of wishes.
- At the Fairy Forest, in Fort William, Scotland, people travel from all over the world to leave letters, drawings, prayers, and gifts for personal and planetary healing.
- Every year at Chinese New Year, people travel to a banyan tree in Lam Tsuen, Hong Kong, to write wishes on colorful slips of paper and hang them on the tree.
- In Siberia, trees are seen as sacred bridges between heaven and Earth. Traditionally, prayer trees are junipers but can be any type of evergreen.

Invite your neighbors, colleagues, and friends to tie colored cloth ribbons to the tree. Don't tie the ribbons too tightly—leave plenty of room for the tree to continue to grow. Encourage people to be creative and knit, craft, or crochet their own prayer objects. Let this be a tree where the community can gather and share what's in their hearts.

Once you've shown that any tree can be sacred, others may begin to see that all trees are sacred. You become an active participant in our societal journey to reconnection. By bringing the knowledge of the forest back to your community, you reconnect more deeply and inspire others around you to see the world with new eyes. It might not seem like much, but sometimes it doesn't take much to change the course of someone's life. A few moments of sacred connection is all it takes to begin to shed our outer layers and connect to our inner ones.

honor the
old-growth

The trees are calling to each of us. When you get quiet, you will hear your call. It may feel like an unpractical yearning at first, and it takes a lot of courage to answer the call.

Old-growth forests—those that have not undergone any major unnatural changes, such as logging—have really called to me. These are the groves that hold the most wisdom.[8] It's in these ancient untampered-with woods that we can experience our own true wildness. These trees are also in desperate need of our protection, as big corporations that are hungry for access to oil and timber threaten their very existence.[9] They see money in these forests but are blind to their true wealth.

There are ancient tree-beings all around us. Pockets of old-growth forests can still be found across the planet and hold the keys to all life on Earth. If we save them, they will save us. Their medicine will cure our ailments. Their ability to influence water flows and weather patterns will save the planet. And their unbridled wildness will heal our souls.

Old-growth forests store genetic information and are home to species that we have yet to meet and have an intelligence we have yet to comprehend. There are magical potions, species, medicines, and curiosities still to be discovered.

Only 15 percent of the ancient old-growth forests that once covered the earth remain intact.[10] The rest of the original forests of the planet have been cleared, degraded, or fragmented. It takes at least five hundred years for a forest to be considered old-growth. As compared to the long history of the universe, the systematic genocide of old-growth forests has happened suddenly. It started with the onset of agriculture twelve thousand years ago, but a lot of deforestation has happened in the past century—even the past few years.

The first time I heeded the call, I visited the ancient kauri trees on the North Island of New Zealand. Although it involved a long trip across the ocean, I simply could not be dissuaded from going. I had to be among these giant beings, even though I didn't know why. *Te Matua Ngahere* ("father of the forest" in Maori) is a three-thousand-year-old kauri tree (*Agathis australis*) in the Waipoua Forest. To forest bathe among such ancient beings is to enter a mystical world—it's a surreal experience.

Not long after returning from my encounter with the kauri trees, I learned that as part of New Zealand's "family of ancient trees" project, the tallest tree in New Zealand, *Tāne Mahuta*, would have a new "sister tree," *Jomon Sugi*, in Japan. This ancient Japanese cedar resides on Yakushima Island. I knew I had to pay my regards to Jomon Sugi while in Japan. From Kyoto, I took a train, a plane, a taxi, and a ferry to Yakushima Island, and then took a bus, hitchhiked, a walked eleven kilometers to reach this tree. When I finally arrived, I realized that it was not the moment of seeing the tree that mattered, but the journey I took to get there.

It was before hopping the flight to see Jomon Sugi that I first talked with author Llyn Cedar Roberts. I had fallen in love with the book *Speaking with Nature: Awakening to the Deep Wisdom of the Earth*, whichshe cowrote with Sandra Ingerman. She was living in Washington's Hoh Rainforest while writing the book, and I knew in my heart that I needed to visit the Hoh, the largest temperate rainforest in the world. I asked her for advice on how to visit the Hoh and was pleasantly surprised when she responded and agreed to talk.

The day after the trek to Jomon Sugi, I received an eleven-minute voicemail from Llyn. She realized that she was meant to meet me in the Hoh Forest, and that the autumnal equinox was the exact right time. She knew that the Hoh was connecting us for some divine purpose that we could not predict. We had to show up for it in full integrity. And we did. Llyn shared her sacred practices, her special home, and the wisdom she has received from thirty years of this work.

Nothing's been quite the same since leaving the Hoh. Before, I may have questioned some of it—How do I know if a tree is *really* calling to me? But now I trust in the deep wisdom of the unfolding. Each time I follow my intuition to visit an ancient forest, I have been propelled further on my own journey, the great unfolding of my own life.

It's not too late. Now is the time to honor the old-growth forests that remain. Hold them in your heart. Pray for them. Pay your respects to them. Treat them like the elders of your own family. Feel the connection in your heart. The work of saving the earth is actually work that we need to do to save ourselves. Now is the time to save ourselves from our destructive slumbers and wake up to the magic that surrounds us.

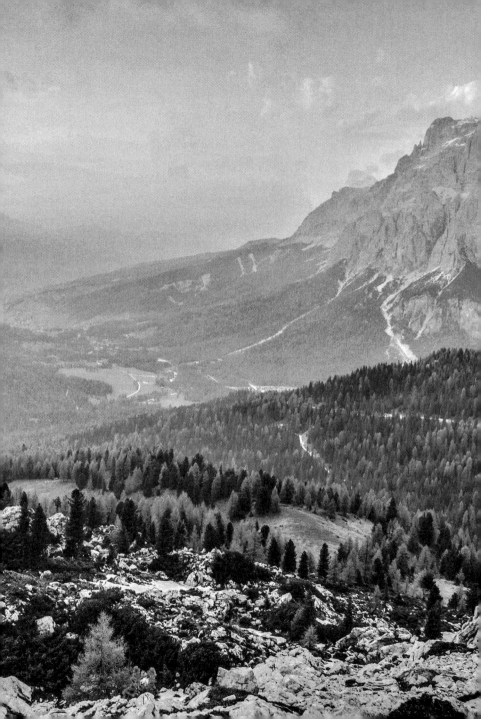

heal the planet

Now you see it. This is the moment. Humans have been on a trajectory of distraction and overconsumption for centuries, and we had to reach the breaking point for the great transformation to begin. We've become completely misaligned—with ourselves and the earth. Now is the time to begin the process of coming back to ourselves and to one another. This is what forest bathing is all about.

All the facts and data around the benefits of being in nature encourage us to step into the forest, where we will discover our own truths. We need space and time to find ourselves. In the forest, we can discover our infinite capacity for love, courage, and creativity.

As you wake up to love, you will also feel pain and sorrow. This is part of the same process—love and pain are two sides of the same coin. Spend time alone and also with a group, because when we are together, we can experience the universality of our feelings and share in our grief and sorrow for the current state of the planet. It's okay to feel the pain and to cry as emotions move through you—it is natural as we open our hearts to Mother Earth.

And then move through the grief. Use grief like a fertilizer to bring about new life. Do something—anything—organize a neighborhood cleanup, plant trees, volunteer your time, and bring people into the forest. As you take part in the healing of our world, you connect to your natural intelligence, your community, and all of life.

Join the largest movement in human history—an era of restoration and regeneration that will change every aspect of our lives. This is the age of learning from nature and living in harmony with all of life. It's impossible to know how many organizations are committed to serving the planet, but there must be millions around the world. This movement defies definition: there are no leaders or manifestos. This global environmental movement also serves social justice and humanitarian efforts. It is a wide-sweeping awakening arising from Earth herself and manifesting through each of us.

Don't worry about doing everything. It's when the task seems so overwhelming that we end up in a state of anxiety, fear, and paralysis. Remember to take care of yourself, love yourself, and enjoy the miracle that is every living thing. The great shift to a life-sustaining society is sprouting up in countless ways. Native and indigenous wisdom-keepers around the globe are sharing their original instructions for living with us and through us. Healers, shamans, and artists among us are coming forward to share their gifts and exude gratitude. As Chief Oren Lyons says, "Two things were told to us [by our ancestors]: to be thankful, so those are our ceremonies, ceremonies of thanksgiving. We built nations around it, and you can, too. And the other thing they said was enjoy life."[11] The more you are truly living in joy, the more aligned you are with the forces of life.

Scientists, designers, and innovators are also creating new ways of generating energy, producing food and clothes, living on the land, and even measuring wealth. Some of these new ways of being hark back to the very old, traditional ways that our ancestors lived.

Even politicians and policymakers around the world are beginning to incorporate indigenous beliefs into laws and give rights to Nature:

- New Zealand's Parliament declared that the country's third-largest river, the Whanganui, has the same legal rights as a person, becoming the first river in the world to be recognized as a living entity. The passing of this bill culminates a 140-year campaign by indigenous groups. The Maori believe that the well-being of the river is directly linked to the well-being of the people.[12]
- Ecuador rewrote its constitution in 2008 to give Nature "the right to exist, persist, maintain, and regenerate its vital cycles."[13]
- Bolivia passed the Law of the Rights of Mother Earth, giving Nature equal rights to humans in 2010. The draft of the new law refers to Pachamama as a living being: "Mother Earth is a dynamic living system comprising an indivisible community of all living systems and living organisms, interrelated, interdependent, and complementary, which share a common destiny."[14]

Earth rights are human rights, for we cannot thrive when we are living out of harmony with our environment. We humans are the caretakers, wild-tenders, and restorers of the Earth. Some of us have always known this, and others of us are just awakening to this knowing that has always been in our hearts. Beyond anxiety, stress, fear, and despair, there is infinite hope, joy, and opportunity. Discover it yourself. This is what you will find when you step into the forest.

Further Reading

Ackerman, Diane. *A Natural History of the Senses*. New York: Vintage, 1991.

Blackie, Sharon. *If Women Rose Rooted: The Journey to Authenticity and Belonging*. London: September Publishing, 2016.

Buhner, Stephen Harrod. *The Secret Teachings of Plants: The Intelligence of the Heart in the Direct Perception of Nature*. Rochester, VT: Bear & Company, 2004.

Emerson, Ralph Waldo. "Nature," in *Nature and Selected Essays*. New York: Penguin, 1982.

Estés, Clarissa Pinkola. *Women Who Run with the Wolves: Myths and Stories of the Wild Woman Archetype*. New York: Ballantine Books, 1992.

Goodall, Jane. *Seeds of Hope: Wisdom and Wonder from the World of Plants*. New York: Grand Central Publishing, 2014.

Hanh, Thich Nhat. *Love Letter to the Earth*. Berkeley, CA: Parallax Press, 2013.

Hawken, Paul. *Blessed Unrest: How the Largest Movement in the World Came into Being and Why No One Saw It Coming*. New York: Viking, 2007.

Ingerman, Sandra, and Llyn C. Roberts. *Speaking with Nature: Awakening to the Deep Wisdom of the Earth*. Rochester, VT: Bear & Company, 2015.

Kimmerer, Robin Wall. *Braiding Sweetgrass: Indigenous Wisdom, Scientific Knowledge, and the Teaching of Plants*. Minneapolis, MN: Milkweed Editions, 2013.

Kornfield, Jack. *After the Ecstasy, the Laundry: How the Heart Grows Wise on the Spiritual Path*. New York: Bantam Books, 2001.

Li, Qing. *Forest Bathing: How Trees Can Help You Find Health and Happiness*. New York: Viking, 2018.

Macy, Joanna, and Molly Brown. *Coming Back to Life: The Updated Guide to the Work That Reconnects*. Gabriola Island, BC, Canada: New Society, 2014.

Megré, Vladimir. *Anastasia*, Book 1, Ringing Cedars Series. Stateline, NV: Ringing Cedars Press, 2005.

Milton, John P. *Sky Above, Earth Below: Spiritual Practice in Nature*. Boulder, CO: Sentient Publications, 2006.

Nelson, Melissa K. *Original Instructions: Indigenous Teachings for a Sustainable Future*. Rochester, VT: Bear & Company, 2008.

Prechtel, Martin. *Secrets of the Talking Jaguar: Memoirs from the Living Heart of a Mayan Village*. New York: Tarcher/Putnam, 1999.

Roberts, Llyn C. *Shapeshifting into Higher Consciousness: Heal and Transform Yourself and Our World with Ancient Shamanic and Modern Methods*. Alresford, Hampshire, UK: O-Books, 2011.

Snyder, Gary. *Turtle Island*. New York: New Directions Books, 1974.

Williams, Florence. *The Nature Fix: Why Nature Makes Us Happier, Healthier, and More Creative*. New York: W. W. Norton, 2017.

Williams, Terry Tempest. *When Women Were Birds: Fifty-Four Variations on Voice*. London: Picador, 2013.

Wohlleben, Peter. *The Hidden Life of Trees: What They Feel, How They Communicate*. Vancouver, BC: Greystone Books, 2016.

Endnotes

PART 1: BEGIN THE JOURNEY TO RECONNECTION

1. Targum and Rosenthal, "Seasonal Affective Disorder," *Psychiatry (Edgmont)* 5 (May 2008): 31–33.

2. Linnie Marsh Wolfe, ed. *John of the Mountains: The Unpublished Journals of John Muir* (Madison, WI: The University of Wisconsin Press, 1938): 313.

3. Deborah Needleman, "The Rise of Modern Ikebana," *New York Times* (November 6, 2017), www.nytimes.com/2017/11/06/t-magazine/ ikebana-japanese-flower-art.html.

4. In a 2009 study on the therapeutic effects of forest bathing (see www.ncbi.nlm.nih.gov/pmc/articles/PMC2793341).

5. Sarah Sekula, "Forest Bathing: A Walk in the Woods," *Orlando Magazine* (August 2017), www.orlandomagazine.com/Orlando-Magazine/August-2017/Forest-Bathing-A-Walk-in-the-Woods.

6. "An Interview with Forest Medicine and Shinrin Yoku Researcher Dr. Qing Li," *Hiking Research* (November 23, 2012), hikingresearch .wordpress.com/2012/11/23/an-interview-with-forest-medicine-and-shinrin-yoku-researcher-dr-qing-li.

7. www.nami.org/Learn-More/Mental-Health-By-the-Numbers.

8. See E. J. Mundell, "Rise in Child Chronic Illness Could Swamp Health Care," *ABC News* (March 23, 2018), abcnews.go.com/Health/ Healthday/story?id=4507708.

9. "The Growing Crisis of Chronic Disease in the United States," Partnership on Chronic Disease, www.fightchronicdisease.org/sites/ default/files/docs/GrowingCrisisofChronicDiseaseintheUSfact sheet_81009.pdf.

10. Marco Lambertini, "Our Planet Is at Breaking Point. But It's Not Too Late to Save It," *World Economic Forum* (January 5, 2017), www.weforum.org/agenda/2017/01/our-planet-is-at-breaking-point-but-it-s-not-too-late-to-save-it/.

11. Joanna Macy wrote of the Shambala warrior, a Tibetan legend, for *Awakin.org* (July 8, 2002), www.awakin.org/read/view.php?tid=236.

12. To read Eisenstein's essay, see charleseisenstein.net/essays/the-three-seeds.

PART 2: HEED THE CALL OF THE FOREST

1. C. Nautiyal, et al., "Medicinal Smoke Reduces Airborne Bacteria," *Journal of Ethnopharmacology* (December 3, 2007), www.greenmedinfo.com/article/medicinal-smoke-can-completely-eliminate-diverse-plant-and-human-pathogenic-bacteria-air; and A. Mohagheghzadeh et al., "Medicinal Smokes," *Journal of Ethnopharmacology* (November 24, 2006), www.greenmedinfo.com/article/medicinal-smoke-may-have-broad-range-therapeutic-applications-and-benefits.

2. See Marlynn Wei, MD, "5 Ways Stress Hurts Your Body, and What To Do About It," *Psychology Today* (May 7, 2015), www.psychologytoday.com/us/blog/urban-survival/201505/5-ways-stress-hurts-your-body-and-what-do-about-it.

3. Florence Williams, "How Just 15 Minutes of Nature Can Make You Happier," *Time* (February 7, 2017), time.com/4662650/nature-happiness-stress.

4. See Michael Winnick, "Putting a Finger on Our Phone Obsession: Mobile Touches: A Study on Humans and Their Tech," *dscout* (June 16, 2016), blog.dscout.com/mobile-touches.

5. Drake Baer, "Why Data God Jeffrey Hammerbacher Left Facebook to Found Cloudera," *Fast Company Magazine* (April 18, 2013), www.fastcompany.com/3008436/why-data-god-jeffrey-hammerbacher-left-facebook-found-cloudera.

6. Linda Stone, in her November 24, 2014, blog article, "Are You Breathing? Do You Have Email Apnea?" (lindastone.net/2014/11/24/are-you-breathing-do-you-have-email-apnea).

PART 3: CROSS THE THRESHOLD

1. Clinton Ober, Stephen Sinatra, and Martin Zucker, *Earthing: The Most Important Health Discovery Ever!* (Laguna Beach, CA: Basic Health Publications, 2014).

2. This John Burroughs quote is from the article "Mother Earth," which appeared in *Putnam's Monthly & the Critic* in October 1906.

3. For more information, see "How Much Sun Is Good for Our Health?" at www.sciencedaily.com/releases/2017/03/170308083938.htm.

PART 4: MOVE THROUGH INVITATIONS

1. This quote is from *Conversations of Goethe with Johann Peter Eckermann,* originally published in 1836.

2. Hans Gelter, "*Friluftsliv*: The Scandinavian Philosophy of Outdoor Life," *Canadian Journal of Environmental Education* 5 (Summer 2000): 77.

3. R. H. Ulrich, "View Through a Window May Influence Recovery from Surgery," *Science* (April 27, 1984): 420–21.

4. Lauren F. Friedman and Kevin Loria, "11 Scientific Reasons You Should Be Spending More Time Outside," *Business Insider* (April 22, 2016), www.businessinsider.com/scientific-benefits-of-nature-outdoors-2016-4.

5. "Nature. Beauty. Gratitude," recorded lecture by Louie Schwartzberg at *TEDxSF*, www.ted.com/talks/louie_schwartzberg_nature_beauty_gratitude?language=en.

6. Lara Franco, Danielle Shanahan, and Richard Fuller, "A Review of the Benefits of Nature Experiences: More than Meets the Eye," *International Journal of Environmental Research and Public Health* (August 2017): 864.

7. Sandra T. Weber and Eve Heuberger, "The Impact of Natural Odors on Affective States in Humans," *Chemical Senses* 33 (June 1, 2008): 441–47, academic.oup.com/chemse/article/33/5/441/411550.

8. Bahman Aghaie et al., in "Effect of Nature-Based Sound Therapy on Agitation and Anxiety in Coronary Artery Bypass Graft Patients During

the Weaning of Mechanical Ventilation: A Randomised Clinical Trial," *International Journal of Nursing Studies* (April 2014): 526–38.

9. S. O. Kim and B. Shelby, "Effects of Soundscapes on Perceived Crowding and Encounter Norms," *Environmental Management* (July 2011): 89–97.

10. "Get Touchy Feely with Plants: Gently Rubbing Them with Your Fingers Can Make Them Less Susceptible to Disease," *ScienceDaily* (September 12, 2013), www.sciencedaily.com/releases/2013/09/130912203053.htm.

11. Juyoung Lee et al., "Nature Therapy and Preventive Medicine," in *Public Health: Social and Behavioral Health*, ed. Prof. Jay Maddock (2012), www.intechopen.com/books/public-health-social-and-behavioral-health/nature-therapy-and-preventive-medicine.

12. Diana Beresford-Kroeger, "How Trees Can Heal Us," www.treesisters.org/2017–10–04–18–28–09/blog/79-wild-hope-for-a-new-humanity/554-how-trees-can-heal-us.

13. Zoë Schlanger, "Dirt Has a Microbiome, and It May Double as an Antidepressant," *Quartz* (May 30, 2017), qz.com/993258/dirt-has-a-microbiome-and-it-may-double-as-an-antidepressant/.

14. Helen Thompson, "Early Exposure to Germs Has Lasting Benefits," *Nature* (March 22, 2012), www.nature.com/news/early-exposure-to-germs-has-lasting-benefits-1.10294.

15. Paul K. Piff et al., "Awe, the Small Self, and Prosocial Behavior," *Journal of Personality and Social Psychology* 108 (June 2015): 883–99.

16. Researchers Dacher Keltner and Jonathan Haidt define awe as the emotional state of being that straddles the boundary of pleasure and fear.

17. Brenda Bernstein, "The Power of Awe: 5 Proven Benefits to Experiencing Awe in Your Life," *Essay Expert*, theessayexpert.com/the-power-of-awe-5-proven-benefits-to-experiencing-awe-in-your-life.

18. Stuart Wolpert, "Putting Feelings into Words Produces Therapeutic Effects in the Brain; UCLA Neuroimaging Study Supports Ancient Buddhist Teachings," *UCLA Newsroom* (June 21, 2007), newsroom.ucla.edu/releases/Putting-Feelings-Into-Words-Produces-8047.

19. Juyoung Lee et al.

20. See "How a Week of Camping Resets the Body Clock," *Conversation* (April 1, 2013), theconversation.com/how-a-week-of-camping-resets-the-body-clock-16557.

21. Ralph Waldo Emerson, *Nature and Selected Essays* (New York: Penguin Classics, 2016), 25-82.

22. In fact, according to Diana Beresford-Kroeger, 60 percent of all medicines in the world, including those that form the basis of modern pharmaceuticals, come from the forest, and many plants offer cures that we are not yet even aware of. This is another reason why it's so important to maintain the biodiversity in our forests, which contain unlimited cures for human illnesses. Diana Beresford-Kroeger, "How Trees Can Heal Us," interview by Clare Dubois, TreeSisters (October 2017), www.treesisters.org/2017-10-04-18-28-09/blog/79-wild-hope-for-a-new-humanity/554-how-trees-can-heal-us.

23. The quote is from an interview of William Gibson by David Wallace-Wells. See "William Gibson: The Art of Fiction No. 211," *Paris Review* (Summer 2011), www.theparisreview.org/interviews/6089/william-gibson-the-art-of-fiction-no-211-william-gibson.

24. Drake Baer, "How Dali, Einstein, and Aristotle Perfected the Power Nap," *FastCompany Magazine* (December 10, 2013), www.fastcompany.com/3023078/how-dali-einstein-and-aristotle-perfected-the-power-nap.

25. Francesca Gino, "Why Rituals Work," *Scientific American* (May 14, 2013), www.scientificamerican.com/article/why-rituals-work.

PART 5: FIND YOUR TRUE NATURE

1. See Swami et al., "Self-Esteem Mediates the Relationship Between Connectedness to Nature and Body Appreciation in Women, but Not Men," *Body Image* 16 (March 2016): 41–44.

2. Arjun Walla, "Nothing Is Solid & Everything Is Energy: Scientists Explain the World of Quantum Physics," *Collective Evolution* (September 27, 2014),

www.collective-evolution.com/2014/09/27/this-is-the-world-of-quantum-physics-nothing-is-solid-and-everything-is-energy.

3. Steve Taylor, "The Power of Nature: Ecotherapy and Awakening," *Psychology Today* (April 28, 2012), www.psychologytoday.com/blog/out-the-darkness/201204/the-power-nature-ecotherapy-and-awakening.

4. Myke Johnson, "Wanting to be Indian: When Spiritual Turns into Cultural Theft," *Unsettling America: Decolonization in Theory & Practice* (September 20, 2011), unsettlingamerica.wordpress.com/2011/09/20/wanting-to-be-indian.

5. See "Is this Japanese concept the secret to a long, happy, meaningful life?" *World Economic Forum* (August 9, 2017), www.weforum.org/agenda/2017/08/is-this-japanese-concept-the-secret-to-a-long-life/.

PART 6: RETURN WITH YOUR ELIXIR

1. Amy Morin, "7 Scientifically Proven Benefits of Gratitude," *Psychology Today* (April 3, 2015), www.psychologytoday.com/blog/what-mentally-strong-people-dont-do/201504/7-scientifically-proven-benefits-gratitude.

2. John Dewey said in his book *How We Think*, "We do not learn from experience . . . we learn from reflecting on experience." (Boston, MA: D.C. Heath and Co. [1933]: 78.)

3. "Neil deGrasse Tyson's Top Ten Favorite Facts About the Universe," *Washington Post* (December 16, 2007), www.washingtonpost.com/wp-dyn/content/article/2007/12/14/AR2007121400571.html?noredirect=on.

4. Pat McCabe, "Wild Hope for a New Humanity," interview by Clare Dubois, TreeSisters (November 2017), www.soundcloud.com/treesisters/patmccabe-woman-stands-shining-wild-hope-for-a-new-humanity-series.

5. "Do We Underestimate the Power of Plants and Trees?" *BBC News* (November 20, 2015), www.bbc.com/news/science-environment-34849374.

6. Jocelyn Mercado, "The Incredible Hidden Life of Trees," Pachamama Alliance (March 16, 2016), www.pachamama.org/blog/the-incredible-hidden-life-of-trees.

7. Sandra Ingerman, "How to Create a Prayer Tree in Your Local Community," *Huffington Post* (November 16, 2011), www.huffingtonpost.com/entry/community-prayer-tree_b_1091710.html.

8. "What Is an Old-Growth Forest?" *Oregon Wild* (2014), www.oregonwild.org/oregon_forests/old_growth_protection/what-is-an-old-growth-forest.

9. US Forest Service study (www.fs.fed.us/pnw/pubs/pnw_rb197.pdf), according to the World Wildlife Federation (www.worldwildlife.org/threats/deforestation).

10. P. Potapov, et al., "The Last Frontiers of Wilderness: Tracking Loss of Intact Forest Landscapes from 2000 to 2013" *Science Advances* (2017): 3:e1600821, http://www.intactforests.org.

11. Melissa K. Nelson, ed., *Original Instructions: Indigenous Teachings for a Sustainable Future* (Rochester, VT: Bear & Company, 2008).

12. "New Zealand River Legally Granted Same Rights as Humans," *Yale Environment* (March 16, 2017), e360.yale.edu/digest/new-zealand-river-legally-granted-same-rights-as-humans.

13. "Ecuador Adopts Rights of Nature in Constitution," Rights of Nature, therightsofnature.org/ecuador-rights.

14. See "Law of Mother Earth, The Rights of a Planet: A Vision from Bolivia," World Future Fund, www.worldfuturefund.org/Projects/Indicators/motherearthbolivia.html.

About the Author

JULIA PLEVIN is an author, award-winning designer, and the founder of Forest Bathing Club, an international community of individuals seeking to connect to nature as a way to heal themselves, their communities, and the planet. She designs and facilitates transformational nature-connected healing experiences for individuals, communities, and corporations. Her work has been featured across international media outlets, including *The New Yorker*, *Business Insider*, *Outside* magazine, *Fast Company*, *Popular Science*, and on CNN. Julia holds a BA in history from Dartmouth College and an MFA in products of design from the School of Visual Arts. She currently lives among the redwood trees in Northern California and splits her time between the forest and the ocean.

Special Thanks

Infinite gratitude to Pachamama and all the beings who have supported me on this journey. At times it can feel that writing a book is a solitary pursuit, but even when I was all alone, writing from a cold cabin in West Marin, I felt in my heart that I was deeply supported in this work.

First, always, is my family—Mark Plevin, Amy Plevin, and Rebecca Plevin. Thank you for believing in me when I did not believe in myself. Thank you for being my first editor, my best muse, and my best friend, respectively. And Milo the dog for being the best coworker I've ever had. To all my grandparents, especially my late grandfather Gerald Plevin, a high school English teacher, who encouraged my love of whimsical writing from a very young age.

I would like to thank my mentors who appeared out of the woodwork once I stepped into the forest: Llyn Cedar Roberts for sharing her sacred home and infinite wisdom with me. Mark Morey for tending his fire and showing me how to tend mine. Alena Eckelmann and Tateishi Kosho for their open hearts and dedication to the way of En no Gyōja. M. Amos Clifford for following his Earth dreamings and bringing the practice of forest bathing to North America.

Thanks to the team of nature-connected women at Ten Speed Press: Ashley Pierce, Kara Plikaitis, and especially Kelly Snowden for holding a vision for this book before we even met.

And to all those whom I have met along the way—I would not be here without your encouragement. Thank you, my dear friends, muses, teachers, and fellow dreamers, and to my community in the Bay Area and beyond. To Spencer Arnold for encouraging me to host my first forest bath, to Kristine Arth for designing logos for my wild ideas and making me laugh always, and to Lauren Magrisso for keeping me sane and fed during my Thoreau stint in Stinson Beach. Thanks to the members of Forest Bathing Club and everyone who has come along on a forest bath with me.

Thank you to all the trees—the ones still standing and the ones who now have second lives as musical instruments, homes, furniture, and pages of books. It's the trees that make it possible to share ideas and the written word in this way. I have a personal intention to plant as many trees as possible in reciprocity for the opportunity to share this book, and I invite you to do the same.

"If women remember that once upon a time we sang with the tongues of seals and flew with the wings of swans, that we forged our own paths through the dark forest while creating a community of its many inhabitants, then we will rise up rooted, like trees . . . well then, women might indeed save not only ourselves but the world."

—SHARON BLACKIE, *If Women Rose Rooted*

Index

A

air, 92
Akiyam5a, Tomohide, 14, 15
Aristotle, 78, 107
awe, 83

B

biophobia, 29
breathing, 42, 92
Buhner, Stephen Harrod, 120
Burke, Edmund, 125
Burroughs, John, 61

C

cacao, 113
Cambell, John, 78
ceremonies, 111–13
cladoptosis, 84
clothing, 28, 30
cortisol, 16
creativity, 105–7

D

Dali, Salvador, 109
Dewey, John, 139
direct perception, 120
dreams, 109–10

E

Earth
    asking permission from, 59–60
    as energy source, 55, 86
    as feminine force, 2
    giving back to, 57–58
    healing, 151–53
    walking barefoot on, 54–55
    See also Nature; Universe
earth (element), 91
earthing, 55
eating, 100–103
ecotherapy, 117–18
Eisenstein, Charles, 20
elements
    connecting to, 93
    four, 90–93
Emerson, Ralph Waldo, 95
emotions, releasing, 38–39
energy, 61–62
entelechy, 131
essential oils, 76
Estés, Clarissa Pinkola, 1

F

fire, 92–93
food, 100–103
foraging, 101–2
forest bathing
    benefits of, 11, 13–14, 16–17, 21, 151
    as ceremony, 111
    clothing for, 28, 30
    ending, 135
    experiencing, 2
    history of, 14–15, 17
    as journey, 22, 26–29, 36
    location for, 33–35
    meaning of, 13
    as medicine, 6, 16
    modern life and, 15–17

preparing for, 26–31
rewilding and, 2–3
safety and, 29–31
as way of life, 22–23
Forest Bathing Club, 9–10
fractals, 72–73
Friedan, Betty, 9
friluftsliv, 23

G

gekkou yoku, 48
Gibson, William, 108–9
Goethe, Johann Wolfgang von, 73
Goodall, Jane, 99
gratitude, 53, 136–37
grief, 151–52
guideposts, 125–26

H

haiku, 14, 106
hākuturi, 60
Hammerbacher, Jeffrey, 41
head, alignment of, 48–49
heart
    chakra, 120
    following, 120–21
    strengthening, 119
herbs, burning, 30–31
huaca, 127–29

I

ikebana, 14–15, 106
ikigai, 131
intentions, setting, 45–47

interbeing, 1, 52
invitations, moving through, 69

J

Jomon Sugi, 148–49
journaling, 26–27
journeying, 129

K

Kawase, Toshiro, 15
Kornfield, Jack, 47, 133

L

letting go, 84–85
Li, Qing, 16
listening, 77
looking up, 83
love
    pain and, 151
    self-, 116–18
Lyons, Chief Oren, 18, 152

M

ma, 71
Macy, Joanna, 19
mandalas, 107
Mandelbrot, Benoit, 72
Mayan calendar, 47
McCabe, Pat, 140–41
medicine, discovering, 130–33
moonrise bathing, 48
Muir, John, 14
mycorrhizae, 143–44

N

napping, 108–10
Nature
  disconnection from, 6–7, 8, 18–20
  guideposts of, 125–26
  as healer, 75, 79, 102
  importance of, 17
  learning from, 10, 44, 101, 123–26
  maintaining connection with, 140–41
  as mirror, 123
  rights for, 153
  signposts of, 124
  wisdom of, 123
  See also Earth; Universe
negative ions, 79, 81
Nhat Hanh, Thich, 52, 55
Nin, Anaïs, 105–6

O

offerings, giving, 57–58
old-growth forests, 147–49
Ortega y Gassett, José, 42

P

peace trees. See prayer trees
permission, asking, 59–60
Pert, Candace, 38
phones, turning off, 41–42
phytoncides, 15, 79, 80
Pollock, Jackson, 126
potential, realizing, 131
prana, 63
prayer, 52–53
prayer trees, 145–46
presence, practicing, 43–44
prophecies, 20–21
protection, 29–31
psychoterratica, 6

Q

qi, 63
qigong, 63

R

Rātā, 60
reflection, 138–39
relaxing, 39, 72–73
rewilding, 2–3
rhythm, 86–87
rituals, 111–13
Roberts, Llyn Cedar, 62, 110, 127, 149
Roszak, Theodore, 118
Rumi, 67

S

sacred objects, 30, 127–29
sacred spots, 97–99
SAD (seasonal affective disorder), 7
safety, 29–31, 53
Schwartzberg, Louie, 76
self-love, 116–18
senses
  number of, 78
  reinvigorating, 75–78
shadows, 36–37
shaking, 38–39
shakti, 63
Shambala warriors, 19
sharing, 71, 139, 143–44
shinrin-yoku, 14
Shugendō Buddhism, 15, 45, 54
Siberian Mark, 110
signposts, 124
silence, walking in, 70–71
singing, 88–89
smell, sense of, 76–77
soil bacteria, 79, 81
Steinbeck, John, 83
stress, releasing, 38–39
sun, greeting, 65–67

T

talking piece, 71, 139
Tāne Mahuta, 60, 148
taste, sense of, 78
technology, disconnecting from,
    41–42
Te Matua Ngahere, 60, 148
Thoreau, Henry David, 13
threshold, crossing, 51
Tokin, B. P., 80
touch, sense of, 77
tree calling sense, 78
tree qigong, 63–64
trees
    connecting with, 63–64
    conversing with, 94–95
    energy of, 61–62
    interconnections between, 143–44
    prayer, 145–46
    as symbols, 124
Tyson, Neil deGrasse, 49, 140
Tzolk'in, 47

U

Universe
    expansion of, 106
    size of, 49
    studying, 48
    See also Earth; Nature

V

vision, 76

W

wabi-sabi, 14
walking
    barefoot, 54–55
    in silence, 70–71
    tree breaths, 62
water, 91, 140–41
Watts, Alan, 48

Williams, Terry Tempest, 37
wisdom, 120, 123
wishing trees. *See* prayer trees

Y

Yamabushi, 15, 45–65
Yong Quan, 55

Published in the United States by Ten Speed Press, an imprint of the
Crown Publishing Group, a division of Penguin Random House LLC, New York.

www.crownpublishing.com

www.tenspeed.com

Ten Speed Press and the Ten Speed Press colophon are
registered trademarks of Penguin Random House LLC.

Photo credits:

Cover image © Cameron Davidson/Gallery Stock; page ii © Corey Hendrickson/Gallery
Stock; pages 12 and 68–69 © Florian Stern/Gallery Stock; page 41 © Christopher Simpson/
Gallery Stock; page 56 © Greg Girard/Gallery Stock; page 74 © Florian Groehn/Gallery
Stock; page 82 © David Reinfeld/Gallery Stock; page 96 © Ken Rhodes/Gallery Stock; page
104 © Craig Cameron Olsen; page 122 © James Leighton/Gallery Stock; pages 134–135 ©
Frank Kappa/Gallery Stock; page 142 © Stefan Kuhn/Gallery Stock; pages vi, 4–5, 24–25, 32,
50–51, 114–115, and 150 © Gallery Stock.

Library of Congress Cataloging-in-Publication Data

Names: Plevin, Julia, 1987- author.

Title: The healing magic of forest bathing : finding calm, creativity,
    and connection in the natural world / by Julia Plevin.

Description: First edition. | New York : Ten Speed Press, 2018. |
    Includes bibliographical references and index. ⸒

Identifiers: LCCN 2018026852

Subjects: LCSH: Nature—Psychological aspects. | Nature, Healing power of. |
    Forests and forestry—Health aspects.

Classification: LCC BF353.5.N37 .P54 2018 | DDC 155.9/1—dc23

LC record available at https://lccn.loc.gov/2018026852

Hardcover ISBN: 978-0-399-58211-0

eBook ISBN: 978-0-399-58212-7

Printed in the United States

Design by Leona Chelsea Legarte

10 9 8 7 6 5 4 3 2

First Edition

SUSTAINABLE
FORESTRY
INITIATIVE

Certified Sourcing
www.sfiprogram.org
SFI-01681

The text paper is SFI certified.